This Crazy Vegan Life

A Prescription for an Endangered Species

Christina Pirello

HOME

A HOME BOOK
Published by the Penguin Group
Penguin Group (USA) Inc.
375 Hudson Street, New York, New York 10014, USA
Penguin Group (Canada), 90 Eglinton Avenue East, Suite 700, Toronto, Ontario M4P 2Y3, Canada
(a division of Pearson Penguin Canada Inc.)
Penguin Books Ltd., 80 Strand, London WC2R 0RL, England
Penguin Group Ireland, 25 St. Stephen's Green, Dublin 2, Ireland (a division of Penguin Books Ltd.)
Penguin Group (Australia), 250 Camberwell Road, Camberwell, Victoria 3124, Australia
(a division of Pearson Australia Group Pty. Ltd.)
Penguin Books India Pvt. Ltd., 11 Community Centre, Panchsheel Park, New Delhi—110 017, India
Penguin Group (NZ), 67 Apollo Drive, Rosedale, North Shore 0632, New Zealand
(a division of Pearson New Zealand Ltd.)
Penguin Books (South Africa) (Pty.) Ltd., 24 Sturdee Avenue, Rosebank, Johannesburg 2196, South Africa

Penguin Books Ltd., Registered Offices: 80 Strand, London WC2R 0RL, England

While the author has made every effort to provide accurate telephone numbers and Internet addresses at the time of publication, neither the publisher nor the author assumes any responsibility for errors, or for changes that occur after publication. Further, the publisher does not have any control over and does not assume any responsibility for author or third-party websites or their content.

First edition: December 2008

Library of Congress Cataloging-in-Publication Data

Pirello, Christina.
    This crazy vegan life : a prescription for an endangered species / Christina Pirello.— 1st ed.
        p.   cm.
    Includes index.
    ISBN 978-1-55788-538-8
    1. Veganism.   2. Vegan cookery.   I. Title.
    TX392.P565 2008
    641.5'636—dc22   2008030715

PRINTED IN THE UNITED STATES OF AMERICA

10   9   8   7   6   5   4   3   2   1

PUBLISHER'S NOTE: The recipes contained in this book are to be followed exactly as written. The publisher is not responsible for your specific health or allergy needs that may require medical supervision. The publisher is not responsible for any adverse reactions to the recipes contained in this book.

Most Home books are available at special quantity discounts for bulk purchases for sales promotions, premiums, fund-raising, or educational use. Special books, or book excerpts, can also be created to fit specific needs. For details, write: Special Markets, Penguin Group (USA) Inc., 375 Hudson Street, New York, New York 10014.

This Crazy Vegan Life

To Robert, for his vision and his unconditional love in this crazy vegan life.

To Michele, who is the glue that holds it all together.

Contents

Introduction

I have been lucky with circumstances in my life. I decided who I would be in the world, worked at it and now I live that life. I adopted a vegan lifestyle about twenty-five years ago so that I could live more healthfully and compassionately; making my best effort to do no harm in my days. I discovered that it's everyone's birthright to live this way, but for some reason we don't. So here we are.

With the help of the advice in this book, you're going to lose weight, get fit, get healthy, look young, age magnificently, be nice to the planet and fundamentally rethink your life. It sounds like a lot, so don't panic. You don't need to be a rocket scientist to do all this but you'll be a genius if you do. You are going to choose brilliant health by eating delicious food and moving your body. You will become a healthy human.

What does that mean exactly? Before you read on, take a minute to do a little personal inventory. How do you feel right now? Can you honestly say that you feel vital and strong? Could you feel better? Do you even know what that means to wake up each day full of vigor, eager to meet the challenges and embrace the opportunities that await you?

Now think about your world. When you're at the local mall, how many of the people you see are truly vital, alert and physically fit? How many have clear eyes, firm, glowing skin, gorgeous hair and a body of normal size? Not many, sadly.

As humans, we have taken ourselves so far from what is natural that we don't know what natural is anymore. We think it's normal to feel tired, lethargic, to have aches, pains, bumps, lumps, bulges, dots, spots and hair in places we didn't think possible and no hair where we want it! We think it's normal to walk with hunched shoulders, head low, guts hanging over our pants, "muffin tops" spilling over our jeans, our hair as lackluster as our skin. What appears to be normal is not how it should be.

Eating food that is not fit for humans carries a hefty price tag; and we are paying it, with tired, achy, overweight, sick, weak bodies and foggy minds. Now, before you close the book and say nuts to her and her attitude; who is she to tell me how to live my life, I'll tell you who. I am one of you. I was where you probably are and I changed completely and rethought everything. And if I can do it, so can you! Like me, you have to have to accept no more excuses; no more bull—from yourself and from others. You have to change the way you think and act.

You've picked up this book for a reason—and it's the best first step you can take to a new life. You can become one of the many people living and breathing a new life, changing your world and the world around you—one broccoli spear at a time, so to speak.

I was on the phone with my publisher, mentor and friend, John Duff, when this book took on life. While we were talking about my next project, the success of the South Beach Diet came up. John said, "Any plan works if you do it." Truer words were never spoken. But that led us to a discussion about the need to rethink what we know about health, weight loss, aging and fitness. Because even with all the nutritional, weight-loss and fitness programs out there, as a nation we are growing less healthy, less fit and fatter.

As a vegan, I can tell you that what you will read in these pages works—if you commit. As a teacher/advocate of healthy vegan cooking I agonize over the fact that many people listen to what I say and agree that it makes sense. But there is a huge disconnect between hearing, understanding—and doing. So I decided to put it all into this book, which demands a rethinking of everything.

This book will guide you to a lifetime of vitality, graceful aging and, yes, your ideal weight, but *you* will have to be the one to commit to real change. Before you quickly place this book back on the shelf because it's scary vegan stuff and what you're looking for is some magic bullet, I want you to understand something: To make the change needed to live a healthy life, free of the aches and pains we consider normal; to remain vital and fit; to age gloriously, not as a burden on society; to have beautiful skin, hair, nails and a body that you love...you need to change how you nourish yourself. That is where the commitment part comes in—and that is, in fact, the magic bullet.

I once studied with a brilliant Japanese philosopher, Michio Kushi, who said that it was easier for people to change their life partners than it was for them to change their food. You may laugh; I did. But then he explained that our food is who we are, right down to the cellular level. We literally are what we eat. Look around and you will see irrefutable evidence of that fact. Think Frank Perdue: You may laugh, but see what I mean? So when I say that committing to the idea of this book involves change, I am talking serious change here. I am talking a big 180. But it's time...seriously.

We are in trouble. We are becoming more and more unhealthy, with disease occurring at much younger ages and reaching epidemic proportions, from diabetes and osteoporosis to cancer and heart disease. And fat? It's time to own up to how truly important our food choices are to our day-to-day well-being and how truly important food choices and exercise are to living long, healthy, productive lives. It's time to move our fat butts, step up and take action. And it ain't about skinless chicken breasts or opting for a bucket of thighs just because there are "no trans fats added" now! This is the real deal, kids. It's time to stop the madness, get off the spiral of unhealthy food, followed by pharmaceuticals, followed by disability...and a bad ending to your personal story.

We're all tired of the screaming headlines, articles, books and talk shows about how easy it is to lose weight and stay healthy for life. If it was so easy, everybody would do it and we would all stop talking about it. I've been known to rant at the television when I watch those ads or infomercials touting the easy and dramatic results achieved by one or two people—with the rest of the country in the "results may vary" fine-print disclaimers. The only result that doesn't vary is that these people are taking your money and leaving you still fat and unhealthy. I say enough already!

In my youth I was athletic, active and happy but always a bit bigger than I should have been—what we might have referred to euphemistically as a "big-boned" girl. I'd tried most of the popular diets from Weight Watchers to the cabbage soup diet but my weight yo-yo'd until I had my own quarter-life crisis. I was diagnosed with a terminal form of leukemia and told that I had mere months to live. I believe that my diagnosis, while shocking, was the result of a lifetime of choices I had made, which resulted in my degenerating health. It's a long story, but the condensed version is that I grew up in an Italian household that lived for food. My mother was always in the kitchen, always at the stove. Food was our answer for everything—the good and the bad. Had a tough day? Eat! Got great grades? Eat! Just showed up in the kitchen because you're bored? Eat! You get the picture. I grew up, eating for every occasion and for no occasion.

My mother, a most amazing cook, insisted that every meal be cooked from scratch and that the family sit together at the table. Her passion for food made from fresh ingredients was rivaled only by her passion for fitness and the environment (long before it was cool). As she and I cooked together or walked to the market together (to be fit and save resources), she lectured me about all things healthy.

By the time I left home, I was sick of it all—the shopping, the gardening, the recycling, the lectures. I became a junk food vegetarian living on sugar, snacks and soda, with every intention of leaving my kitchen days behind. When I got sick, a friend introduced me to Robert Pirello, who calmly but firmly told me that my food choices were directly contributing to my imminent demise and that if I rethought my food, I could recover my health. I know; I know; it's hard to believe—a little ridiculous at the time. Trust me when I say that no one was more skeptical than I was. But I could also hear my mother's voice in my head and I remembered how often she and my grandmother used common food ingredients to cure what ailed us as kids. Maybe it wasn't so nuts after all. With Robert as my guide, I fell in love with this crazy vegan macrobiotic diet and the man who taught me the tricks I would need to survive—literally. I recovered my health in about fourteen months and life was great, stretched out before me with a new viewpoint and a spectacular man.

But not so fast; there's a bit more story after the "…and they lived happily ever after" part. As the years passed and my consciousness and awareness of the power of food grew and changed, I still struggled with my weight, a bit of a surprise considering that everyone I met who was into macrobiotics was rail thin. Save for the time I was sick, I carried just enough excess me around to be well, excessive.

When I began my macrobiotic practice, training and fitness were some of the last things on my mind. Surviving took top priority, as it should have.

I had always been fit; weight training was like breathing for me. I swam competitively in college, but with my diagnosis, my lifestyle changed completely as I walked away from the foods that had contributed to making me sick and left my beloved gym for more "natural" forms of exercise. So from 1984 until 2002, I told myself that this was just how it was; that I was lucky to be alive; that it was my genetic makeup to be "voluptuous." The truth was, I was heavier than I should have been and not as fit as I should have been. I ate too many sweets, albeit healthy ones. I did at-home yoga workouts in an attempt to stay in shape and remain "energetically balanced." I could touch my nose to my knees, but I couldn't run a quarter mile if I had a gun to my head.

My recovery from cancer through a macrobiotic approach to eating opened a whole new world to me, and an understanding of food that I did not imagine existed. My introduction to the concepts of Chinese medicine, natural food and my own studies of conventional nutrition came together to create a new respect for how food choices have an impact on health.

But I had a big disconnect of my very own. I lost sight of the importance of exercise in a healthy life and operated under the delusion that eating well was enough. I was wrong, so I got reconnected right quick, which is why I know that you can, too.

It started in the director's booth. We were filming my fifth season of *Christina Cooks*. I was sitting with the director, watching the "dailies" (the tape of what we had shot that day) when it hit me: I was fat. Granted, they say that the camera adds ten pounds, but I wasn't about to start kidding myself even though I thought I was carrying my excess weight quite well. I wasn't obese, but fatter than I should be. It occurred to me that my little at-home yoga workouts weren't, well, working. I needed more, and that hard look at my body on television did the trick.

And so I did it—I lost weight and got fit. I started by finding a personal trainer. (I know that not everyone has that luxury, but I have a solution for that, too.) And yes, I still work with him to this day, maintaining a level of fitness that I thought was long gone. I work hard and cook my own natural meals with care and attention. But making the change was just as hard for me as it is for everyone else.

I had the cooking thing down pat. I knew what to eat, how to prepare it and how much to eat. But when I started looking closely at every aspect of my life, I realized that I was eating dessert like it was going out of style.

I rationalized this because they were "healthy" sweets. Plus, my schedule of teaching, appearances, travel and running my business had led me to a life of snacking on top of my meals. So while I *knew* what to do, I surely was not doing it. I was still making healthy vegan choices, all appropriate for me, but in excess...and I paid the price in pounds. Now, only I could make that change; make that commitment—just do it.

I have never looked back. And as long as my body holds out, I will never take fitness for granted again. For me, staying fit means so much more than how I look on television. What began as pure vanity has grown into a commitment to health on a new plane.

Now, with what I know, I watch the news and wonder why we are not demanding better information, clearer facts about food and our health. Why is it so hard for us to make the connection between food and its impact on our day-to-day vitality? Why do we not understand that food is powerful enough to cure even the most serious of illnesses, let alone help us achieve our ideal weight? And then something became clear: We have very few examples of that power. It's not what we see in commercials, advertisements and on talk shows. We don't grow up with that thinking ingrained in us. We see people who look fit and healthy chowing down on burgers and fries, sodas and chocolate brownies. We somehow keep missing the truth. When *we* eat those things, we can't see past our fat bellies to our toes.

In this book, I will lay it all out for you. No more excuses. It's do or die for so many of you. Don't you want to feel better, look better and not worry so much? Don't you want to enjoy delicious food and know that it is really nourishing you...and that you don't need to feel guilt at every bite? Don't you want to leave a lighter footprint on the planet? Don't you want to live with compassion? Don't you want the world to be a better place for you having been here?

I'll tell you how I did it: with whole vegan food and cooking and working with Anthony Molino, my friend, trainer and on those days when I can't imagine exercising, my conscience. I have never been pushed to my physical and mental limits as I have with Anthony and I have never felt more excited to work out as I do with his guidance. With his gentle nudging, I trained for and completed my first triathlon at age fifty-one. There is nothing like testing your limits, seeing how much you can really do, pushing yourself as far as you can go and feeling the results—strength, focus, vitality, easy sleep, stamina...and did I mention that I lost thirty-eight pounds?

I'd like to say that it will be easy, but that would just be marketing…and we have been marketed to and brainwashed enough. Some things will be a snap (like *eating* delicious food), but some of what it takes to achieve your ideal weight and regain your health will require commitment and discipline—and some sweat. I believe that people would love to do what is best for their health, but in all the confusion of conflicting information, they are not sure exactly what that is. Most important, they don't know how to actually get started.

So here we are…at the beginning of your journey and the continuation of mine. But it doesn't end with the purchase of this book. I would not be where I am (on so many levels) without the support of others and I would not leave you in the cold either. With *This Crazy Vegan Life* as your guide, you can realize your physical potential, lose weight, live a compassionate life and leave the world a better place. Not a bad deal for a modest initial investment, is it?

See you in the kitchen…or the gym…or both!

Christina
www.christinacooks.com

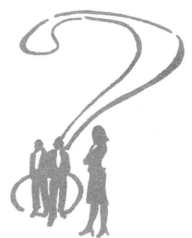

1

How Did We Get into This Mess, Anyway?

American consumers have no problem with carcinogens, but they will not purchase any product, including floor wax, that has fat in it.　　　　　　　— DAVE BARRY

What's not to love about good food? It's nourishing and sensual. It brings people together around the communal or family table. And, not insignificantly, it keeps us alive. But the food of legend, the foods of the harvest table, the ambrosia and nectar of the gods bears little resemblance to what we call food today. In fact, I hardly recognize some of what we eat as food.

ANCIENT HISTORY

We are evolutionarily programmed to eat and rest as much as we can. Seriously, I mean it. When foods like fat and sugar were not abundant and hunting and gathering was an exhausting necessity, we ate and rested to preserve our very lives. Well, I don't know about you, but hunting and gathering are far from exhausting these days—unless finding a parking spot at the supersized market for your supersized car counts. Hunting has become a sport (don't get me started…) and not a necessity. But while things have changed a lot in the past ten thousand years, our basic drive to find food and eat it wherever and whenever we can is still the same. Evolution is a very, very slow process—and, as you'll soon discover, rapid advances in science and technology and rampant commercialism have wreaked havoc with nature's ever evolving plan.

Modern History

Fast forward ten thousand years or so to the middle of the twentieth century when domestic life as we knew it changed forever as one of the many consequences of World War II. With the close of the war we witnessed the beginning of the consumer convenience society that has evolved into the way we live today. (I don't mean to skip over that rather critical period known as the Industrial Revolution, when things really started to heat up what with the abandonment of the primarily rural lifestyle, but for most us what happened at the turn of the last century doesn't feel so relevant.) Events and evolution of the last two generations are fresh in our minds and history books. During the war, women began working outside the home for the first time en masse to keep the country going while all the able-bodied men were overseas. At the war's end, women had realized that there was life beyond the front door. After the Ozzie and Harriet–esque 1950s when it seemed that everyone got a car and moved to the suburbs, we entered the turbulent 1960s and when we emerged from the fog of…well, whatever, women had pretty much abandoned the kitchen, which had been the center of the lives of their mothers and grandmothers. At the same time we were experiencing a dramatically altered economic climate that saw the two-income family as a "necessity" and not a luxury. Money didn't seem to go as far and with the end of the Vietnam War, our mortality really dawned on us and we wanted stuff: lots and lots of stuff. So, all of a sudden (at least in evolutionary terms) we were living in a fast-paced world with lots of labor-saving conveniences, but with no time to stop and smell the roses—or to bake a cake from scratch. And while these observations might be something of a sweeping generalization, home life definitely changed.

Before I incur the wrath of every woman with a feminist bone in her body, let me clarify: I am not saying that women should have no higher ambition than to get a three-course dinner on the table every night, but when we stopped cooking, stopped eating freshly prepared meals at home and stopped coming together around the family table, it was not coincidental that our health began to decline. And one of the last nails in the coffin of our health came with the introduction of convenience foods: canned vegetables, packaged mixes, TV dinners. (And I don't even need to get into the proliferation of fast food restaurants...they were and are, the last nail. Much more about that later.)

WE GET BY WITH A LITTLE HELP FROM OUR FRIENDS

When we stopped "cooking from scratch," somebody had to step in to fill the void as our stoves turned cold and pots and pans gathered dust. And their names read like a list of old friends and relatives: Sarah Lee, Betty Crocker, Aunt Jemima, Uncle Ben, the Pillsbury Doughboy, Cap'n Crunch, Chef Boyardee, Dinty Moore, Oscar Meyer, Mrs. Paul and the friendly and handsome Gorton's Fisherman. And let's not forget Wendy, Denny, Arby or our favorite neighbors, the McDonalds.

To put it bluntly, I think that what the food industry is doing nowadays is criminal. I wish there were a nicer, kinder, more compassionate way to say it. I don't like to be critical of our friends and relatives, even if they exist only in the minds of marketers. Advertising seduces us to eat more and more food, bigger and bigger portions, more and more often. Day after day, you see ads for fast food, junk food, restaurants, frozen food, supermarkets and snacks, all designed to entice us to buy and eat more. Is no one seeing the truth behind the ads? You see slim, fit people sucking down soda, gobbling burgers, chicken nuggets, French fries, candy, chips, cakes and cookies, while they sit in front of the television or play video games. They are all gorgeous, healthy-looking and not *for one second* concerned about the calories, saturated fats, chemicals and additives in their food. Their faces border on orgasmic delight as they eat foods that are so inappropriate for humans that if they in fact, ate those foods, they would look more like the schlubs you see at the mall than the models and actors that they are! Trust me; these slim, gorgeous specimens of humanity are not gorging themselves on that food. I'm not even sure that you can call it food. Michael Pollan, author of *The Omnivore's Dilemma*, describes it the best in his book *In Defense of*

Food when he calls much of what we eat today "food-like substances," with little or nothing to do with food in its whole, natural state.

Q.O.Q.

But we buy into the propaganda and eat and eat and eat less and less natural food. The bigger the combo of burger, soda and fries, the happier we seem to be (or so it appears in the ads). Seriously, do we need a burger that is so big, so disgustingly fatty, covered with cheese, bacon and fattening sauce that it has 1,420 calories and 107 grams of fat? Are we really so crazed with the idea of getting the most for our money—the most fat, the most calories; the most damage to our waistlines, our hearts and to the planet that we've forgotten all about Q.O.Q.: Quality Over Quantity?

Don't Confuse Me with the Facts

If you're looking for a lifeline from the health sciences, you're just as likely to drown in the confusion created by study after study, with results mind-bogglingly different from one another. No wonder we don't know what to do half the time.

Why is the information that you read today so wildly different from last week's "revealing" new study? It is simply because nutrition and its effects on human health are nearly impossible to calculate. To do a really good study you need human subjects, and humans are very hard to control. (Rats are easier to control but they aren't humans…and it's just plain mean to use them in studies so we can figure out how to eat.) How we digest what we eat is unique to each person. How, what, when and why we eat is unique to each of us, too. Left to our own devices, how we measure the amount of food we eat is usually less than accurate. Chewing (or not), what food combinations we choose…every aspect from the preparation to the ingestion to the digestion is a variable. More than one-third of all people underestimate how much inappropriate food they consume and nearly that same number of people overestimate how much appropriate food they eat. Survey after survey shows that people believe they are eating healthy food because they know about it. Not the same thing, but a lovely delusion, I suppose.

However, the biggest problems lie with the studies themselves, in my humble opinion. The largest health studies ever conducted, those that are

considered to be the gold standards of studies of health and human behavior, including the Nurses' Study and the Women's Health Initiative, seem to
have one basic flaw. These studies may tweak a nutrient here or there—eat
less fat or more antioxidants; reduce the carbohydrates or increase the protein—but the inclusion of processed foods, sugars, meat, dairy and poultry,
which are the main ingredients of the Standard American Diet (SAD), are
left largely undisturbed. By studying the effects of diet on typical Americans, the nutrition scientists must study the subjects eating in their typical
way. With the dietary patterns tinkered with rather than radically over-
hauled, is it any wonder that the results are less than revealing? What I am
saying is this: What these studies show us, quite clearly, is that the Standard
American Diet cannot be made healthier unless it is dramatically altered.
You can't simply change up from chicken breasts to skinless chicken breasts
(while leaving most processed food in place) and see dramatic shifts in the
health of a society. You cannot simply have a study group reduce their intake of
chips, cups of coffee or soda and expect to see results that are impressive.
In order to see and experience the power of diet change, we have to change
our eating patterns more dramatically and compare them, as in the Adventist Health Study, where standard eating patterns were compared to those
of the largely vegetarian group the Seventh-day Adventists. This revealing
study compared vegetarian eating and a more meat-based diet. The results
were impressive, showing that vegetarian people lived longer, healthier lives
by a large percentage. And while this study also took into account the fact
that Seventh-day Adventists also do not smoke or drink alcohol, the results
speak for themselves, with Seventh-day Adventist men living 8.9 years longer than others and women 7.5—and that was just in the state of California.

And then there's Dr. T. Colin Campbell, whose groundbreaking book,
The China Study, is a must-read for anyone looking to change their health.
Not only an in-depth study of the effects of dietary patterns on disease,
this book discusses our nutritional confusion and its link to powerful food
lobbies and opportunistic scientists (like those who take money from corporations and then not surprisingly reveal results that favor the funding
company). Dr. Campbell proposes that we are confused by study results
because that is just what marketers and lobbyists want us to be. He says
that the only way to improve health and prevent disease is to "redefine
what we think of as good nutrition." In other words, stop playing with the
details of America's standard way of eating and hoping for better results.

We must change food to change health. Dr. Campbell talks extensively about the connections between our daily food choices and their effects on disease prevention and treatment. Not a dieter's guidebook, *The China Study* cuts through the confusion of so many conflicting studies and comes to the conclusion that is never reached by other studies: We must eat less food and it needs to be whole, natural and from plants.

It's time to stop kidding ourselves with all this tweaking and tinkering, trying to change the way we eat without really making any changes and just bloody change already. Consuming a diet of whole grains, vegetables, beans, fruit, nuts, seeds and healthy fats is the only way to experience health in the way that you want to experience it.

It's time to stop allowing labs and calculations, lobby groups and advertisers trump the influence of the sun, earth, wind and water. It's time to stop kidding ourselves and own up to the fact that the key to health lies in the back garden or the local farm market. People who eat whole, natural foods simply enjoy them. Instead of worrying so much about the nuances of every nutrient in each grain of rice, they spend their time enjoying robust good health, generally free of the specter of degenerative disease and other chronic illness. And yes, at the end of the day, as the saying goes, we will all die. No dietary choices can prevent that, but wouldn't it be nice if the time we spend here was without the preconceived expectation of illness and disability? Wouldn't it be lovely if the chronic illnesses that are the norm today were the exception and not the rule? We must change, *really change* the way we eat for that to be the result. We won't need any more confusing studies.

Let's Drop the Big One and See What Happens

Albert Einstein did not actively participate in the creation of the atomic bomb, but he was instrumental in the thinking behind it. His Theory of Relativity includes the concept that a large amount of energy could be released from a small amount of matter. And he was right. Although Einstein considered himself to be a pacifist, when Hitler rose to power in Germany, he wrote a letter to President Roosevelt urging him to build an atomic bomb before Germany did. Many years later, he wrote that his greatest regret in life was having written this letter. He recognized, too late of course, the trouble that science can create when it becomes enamored with its own creativity and its own power. Imagine what this champion of vegetarianism would think if he saw what science, underwritten by the food industry, has done to our food supply in the name of progress.

All kidding and sarcasm aside, if more people realized what was being done to our food supply there would uprisings in the streets with demands for better quality and more stringent safety standards. But instead, we keep entrusting our health and the health of our loved ones to multinational food corporations and their lobbyists, secure in the knowledge that the powers-that-be in Washington won't let anything bad happen to us. Wake up, people! What's happening to our food is the stuff of nightmares.

The New Food Chain

Pesticides, herbicides, antibiotics, growth hormones and genetic modification are all compromising our food, contributing to the obesity epidemic, speeding up the degeneration of our health and putting the health of the planet at risk. These scientific and technological advances are making slaves of us all.

Pesticides

Pesticides, in particular, organotins, found in food and household cleaning products have been shown to cause aberrant fat cell production and to disrupt endocrine and liver function. Why might that be important? Your liver, the largest gland in your body, has many jobs in the work of keeping you healthy, but its main purpose is to metabolize the macronutrients you consume: fat, protein and carbohydrates. If your liver isn't working at its optimum, you'll have a hard time absorbing and efficiently using nutrients. Even with exercise, you'll consistently struggle with your weight. However, some diet gurus would have you believe you are doomed to be fat just because you have eaten or been exposed to pesticides. You are fat because you choose to eat junk, eat too much and don't exercise—not because you clean your house with commercial products. You can choose to change your diet and lifestyle now. And because your body is an amazing organism, unless you have cirrhosis of the liver or some other disease that has scarred that precious gland, you get a brand-spanking-new liver every seven months or so, as it has the ability to regenerate. Eliminate toxins from your body and it won't take long for your body to rejuvenate itself and begin to metabolize food properly.

We pour nearly three billion (that's billion, with a *b*) pounds of pesticides on our food annually. Ironically, we spend millions on commissions to study their effects on health. Shouldn't we instead be trying to figure out a way to use fewer pesticides in the first place? Or better yet, shouldn't we have studied their effects on health before we decided to use them on our food? It seems their thinking is a bit backward, but that's me.

Of course, we do have the option to buy organic foods. These can be more expensive although not as much as you might think. I'd venture to say that if the big food companies seriously committed to grow and manufacture organic products, the prices would drop to those of commercially produced goods... but for the time being, we have to make the choice to pay now, or pay later. The price of eating non-organic food is a lot higher than you might possibly imagine, as health-care costs skyrocket as a result of our rapidly declining health. And with so much disease directly connected to diet and thereby largely preventable, well, you can draw your own conclusion. I don't know about you, but I am tired of my health-care premiums rising because I have to pay for all the people who choose to compromise their health with junk food.

We also have the option of using natural, nonchemical cleaning products, skin care products and cosmetics, and building or remodeling our homes with natural materials... anything to reduce our exposure to toxins. Our level of exposure is so high that our immune systems are fighting with every shred of strength that they have just to maintain. Making better, more natural choices in every aspect of your life will result in a healthier, stronger you and a healthier, stronger planet. Natural versions exist of just about any household or cosmetic product you can name. Mascara? Yes. Toilet bowl cleaner? Yes. Glass Cleaner? Yup. Floor, dish and laundry soap? You bet. Lawn and garden products? Yes. Moisturizers, sunblock, bug repellent, paint, insulation, flooring... every one of them. You do not need to pollute or ingest toxins to be pretty or suave or to have a clean house and gorgeous garden.

The use of pesticides, fertilizers and herbicides is one of the main pollutants of our waterways, causing about 90% of our rivers to test positively for agricultural pollutants (according to the U.S. Geological Survey), with about twenty different pesticides showing up in the average stream. Yuck! And did I mention that 64% of the life in these waterways—edible fish, mollusks and other aquatic organisms—test positive for the same chemicals. Still think fish is a healthy and safe bet for food?

Herbicides

The use of herbicides is also being questioned on the sustainability front. One scary example out of many is the weed killer Roundup, produced by the agri-giant Monsanto. Most of us only think of Roundup as a way to keep weeds out of our lawns (I could segue to a condemnation of the average American lawn and how it is really bad for the environment but that's for another time…), but the truth is darker and more sinister. When the scientists and marketers at Monsanto discovered that farmers were not applying Roundup to maximum levels because they feared killing their crops along with the weeds, Monsanto created genetically engineered versions of corn and soybeans, called Roundup Ready. These seeds could resist their own herbicide, and forced farmers to apply greater and greater amounts for weed control. This raised a huge red flag about the impact of this chemical—and the genetically engineered products—on our environment and, by extension, on us. It hasn't stopped Monsanto, which trudges on, toxic Goliaths trampling on our health and vitality with their poisons, even though they've been sued by farmers who try to grow natural crops and not buy their sterile and pesticide-laden seeds and chemicals. Not surprisingly, Monsanto sponsors ads that show healthy, lively children running through fields of rice and corn, strong, vital and happy, while in fact, children are most deeply affected by pesticides. According to Californians for Pesticide Reform, children are especially vulnerable to the effects of pesticides. Kids are not just mini-adults; they are growing into adults. Their vulnerability to pesticides is due to their greater cell division rates and being in the early stages of organ and immune system development. A 1993 study by the National Research Council of the National Academy of Sciences revealed that children are more susceptible to the long-term effects of low levels of pesticides than adults as well. So for Monsanto and DuPont to use our kids in their commercials for toxic chemicals is a double insult to our intelligence…if we are paying attention and not just buying the crap they are selling. (And that's just pesticides. More about genetic engineering later on.)

Antibiotics

Thirty-five million pounds of antibiotics are used each year in the United States with 70% of them used to prevent disease and promote growth in our livestock. The idea of antibiotic-resistant bacteria among humanity is of great concern. If you are consistently consuming antibiotics (in your steaks, ribs, chicken nuggets and burgers), what do you think will happen should you need an antibiotic to help your body battle a disease? Nothing, that's what! Your body will have developed immunity to these powerful and some-times necessary drugs. This abuse of antibiotics has spurred the evolution of new strains of antibiotic-resistant bacteria. So if you eat meat tainted with these new "super germs" and fall ill, the chances dramatically increase that the antibiotics administered to cure you will fail. Think I'm exaggerating?

A recent test of Tyson chicken by Johns Hopkins Bloomberg School of Public Health showed that 96% of their meat was contaminated by one of these antibiotic-resistant bacteria. Funny...on their homepage, Tyson thanks mothers everywhere for fighting the "good fight" every day getting kids to eat healthy meals and claims that environmental stewardship is at the core of their business philosophy! Too bad that producing healthy chicken meat isn't, since they had to "tweak" their antibiotic-free claim on their label when the Department of Agriculture found out that it, well, wasn't.

And it's not just chicken. According to the People for the Ethical Treat-ment of Animals (PETA), Montana State University beef specialist John Patterson is quoted as saying, "There is no valid scientific evidence that feeding antibiotics to beef cattle causes human health problems." Really? Then I wonder why the U.S. Department of Agriculture (USDA) reported that exposure to just three to five milligrams of inorganic arsenic (its most toxic form), the kind found in antibiotics used in beef and chicken, can cause cancer, dementia, neurological problems and other ailments in humans. Food for thought, to be sure.

Growth Hormones

Growth hormones aren't just for professional athletes! Growth hormones are used in meat and dairy production at incredibly scary levels. Of the 32.5 million cattle slaughtered annually for your dining pleasure, about two-thirds were injected with growth hormones to make them mature more quickly to meet the demand for meat. On top of that, dairy cows are fed a genetically engineered growth hormone called rBGH to increase milk production. The USDA and Food and Drug Administration (FDA) claim that these hormones are safe, but there is growing concern among experts questioning that thinking. It is now believed that eating the meat and drinking the milk of growth-enhanced animals, which contain residues of these hormones, can actually disrupt the normal hormone function in humans, resulting in everything from early onset of puberty to growth aberrations and even certain cancers. They will not make your children run faster or hit harder or pitch amazing speedballs.

Have you looked at our kids lately? They are so much more mature-looking at earlier and earlier ages, reaching puberty far before what is considered normal. We have more boys with "man breasts" and girls who require breast reduction—all can be linked to consumption of growth hormones in food. I don't know about you, but when I walk past our local elementary school, I am in awe of how adult and fully grown these kids look and act. Where do we think that is coming from? Television? In a single generation the proliferation of steroid use has more than quadrupled so we can produce meat faster and cheaper. Well, this is yet another place where fast and cheap is becoming far too expensive.

And if these hormones are designed to make animals mature more quickly, what do you think will happen to you and your kids? If your children are reaching maturity sooner, it stands to reason that they will degenerate sooner, too. So not only are they losing life expectancy from obesity-related illnesses, but they are decaying at a more rapid rate from early maturity. Yikes!

These insidious toxins affect the planet, too. Growth hormones pass through the cows in their manure and contaminate the soil, surface and ground waters, upsetting delicate ecosystems and life forms. High levels of mammal hormones have been found in wild fish as a result of this contamination and are having a profound impact on gender and reproductive capacity of the fish.

The Environmental Protection Agency (EPA) estimates that nearly 95% of the pesticide residues found in the typical American diet is from meat, dairy and poultry products. Fish (again!) can be particularly toxic with incredibly high levels of carcinogens like PCBs and DDT, not to mention heavy metals like mercury, lead and once again, arsenic (yes, like Lucretia Borgia used to kill her husband). And did I mention that none of these toxins are removed in the freezing or cooking processes?

Genetic Engineering: Not Quite What Nature Intended

Would Albert Einstein have a few things to say about this new kid on the block! Genetically modified organisms (GMO) are engineered in a lab, in petri dishes, without the kiss of the sun and the breeze at their inception. The Roundup Ready soy and corn from Monsanto are but two of thousands of examples. Genetic modification also allows for cross-breeding, which is far removed from natural hybridization. For example, genetic material from salmon can be injected into strawberries to make them more resistant to the cold. Well, if a strawberry and salmon were in a bar, they wouldn't hit on each other and make babies. All joking aside, this is a far cry from a farmer taking a red pepper and a yellow pepper to making an orange pepper—and has far greater consequences than a festive-looking salad or stir-fry.

While the food marketers try to sell us on the concept that GM foods improve yield and pest resistance of crops they also insist that these foods will allow for great strides against hunger and malnutrition in the world. Doesn't that just make you get all warm and fuzzy for Monsanto? Not so fast. There is absolutely no independent proof to the claims concerning increased crop yields and better nutrition (except in studies funded by the companies themselves), but there is increasing concern about the safety of these foods. The spread of pesticide-resistant plants, possible toxicity to wildlife and their impact on human health are of paramount concern. So why do it? Increased control over our food supply by monolithic companies like Monsanto and DuPont give them, in fact, the ultimate power over human life, our very survival. (And you thought the oil cartels were evil!) If you think that these companies care for one second about the starving masses of people around the world, think again. Still think organic is not so important? Still think it's just a bunch of old hippie tree-huggers eating granola and fighting "the establishment"? We should be so lucky. Genetically modified foods should scare you witless. And until we know more about the long-term effects of these foods on us and the planet, we should follow the European example of placing a moratorium on the production of such foods.

READ THE LABELS—IF THERE ARE ANY

The U.S. federal government has made labeling a product as containing GMOs a voluntary process. About 75% of processed foods contain genetically modified ingredients and you would never know it, as there is nothing on the label to inform you. Fresh produce is not exempt either, but you can beat them at their game on this one…sort of. You know all those little stickers on fruit that we hate because they are so hard to get off? Well, they are your little decoder as to the safety of the item. Genetically modified fruits and veggies have a five-digit number beginning with the number *8* on that little sticker. Since labeling is voluntary, you'll be hard-pressed to find those little *8*s anywhere; and since GMOs are now considered a part of conventional growing, they can just as easily label the produce with the conventional labels, but look for them and purchase accordingly. (Conventionally grown produce will have a four-digit number and organic produce will have a five-digit number beginning with *9*.) So am I saying that we have a system that serves everyone's best interest except the consumer? Yes, but we do have a system. Now we just need to inform the consumer and demand that it be utilized.

Since just about all the conventionally grown corn and soybean crops in America are genetically modified, it's important to pay attention to what is in your food. Unless products made from soy or corn are organic—soybean oil, soybeans, soy protein, corn syrup, high-fructose corn syrup, corn starch, corn flour and so on—the odds are they're genetically modified. Buying organic is the only way to know that your food is not genetically altered.

GOOD NEWS, BAD NEWS, GOOD NEWS

Is there any good news about the future of our food supply? Yes, well, maybe. For much of the last century, the big industrial agriculture model has been the one to emulate, with more natural styles of growing, producing and processing being cast aside as old-fashioned and inefficient. For those in the big business of agriculture, progress has meant bigger machines, huge corporate farms, more chemicals and higher-tech breeding.

The alternative to this industrialized version of food production is organic production in which food trade increases income, as well as increasing food safety and security. This system would preserve the environment, give farmers fair access to the means needed to produce food and give consumers fair access to pure food at fair prices. These simple principles create the foundation of organic food production and farming, which have the goal of fair, safe and sane food for everybody.

Concern that state levels of certification were not consistent enough to retain the integrity of organic food production were laid to rest when the USDA put research dollars, enforcement and universal standards in place to ensure the continued growth of the organic food movement. As the organic food industry grew from "fresh and local" to global, consumer confidence was paramount.

The result of these many years of work opened the door for the creation of the National Organic Standards Board, whose primary responsibility was to establish national organic standards for the growth and production of safe and pure food. Organic farmers, food producers and retailers, as well as consumer representatives, scientists and environmentalists worked to create the national organic standards that are in place today. And while many organic proponents (myself included) think that the standards could be more stringent and fear further commercialization and eventual compromise of organics, these standards ensure for now that anything carrying an organic label has been grown and produced without the use of chemical pesticides, herbicides and fungicides; without any genetically modified organisms and free of sewage sludge, growth hormones and antibiotics. And yes, there is growing concern that the small family farm will be edged out of the picture completely as organic farms morph into the same type of monolithic Goliaths as their commercial counterparts. When it becomes more profitable for a farmer to sell his land to "McMansion" developers than to grow food, we are in big trouble. But for now, organic standards are your shield against eating substances that do not even resemble food molecules.

Unfortunately, these standards have been also compromised by the passage of an addendum to our national organic standards. The FDA has allowed that any organic food *may* contain any FDA-approved additives and still be considered a certified organic product. That means organic processed foods, like packaged cereals, salad dressings, convenience foods and frozen entrees could contain the very additives that you are trying to avoid. Your produce is still safe…for now. Another reason to consume freshly prepared meals and not rely on packaged or processed foods.

Organics are still your best choices for keeping your children and your own health safe…and makes your battle for a smaller waistline a little more winnable. Just pay attention and skip the processed food aisle. It's back to the adage of shopping in the periphery of the store for the safest and purest of foods.

Organic Meat

Before you plunk down a week's salary for an organic steak, think about it. Sure, there are no steroid growth hormones, no pesticides, herbicides or fungicides. But there is nothing that can be done to minimize the damage done to your body by all that saturated fat and hard-to-digest protein. There is nothing about the organic production of meat, poultry and dairy foods that mitigates the fact that animals are still being slaughtered at genocide-like numbers. And for what? So you can have a steak and then a heart attack? Yuck!

The future of our food is in jeopardy, but it is also in our hands. By choosing to rethink your life and how you live it, by choosing to feed yourself in a healthy and sustainable way that creates personal health *and* planetary health, you can decide what that future will look like.

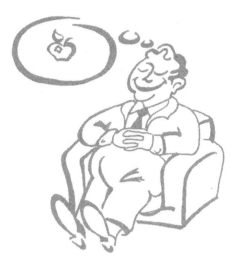

Veganomics: Rethinking Everything

You will never master a problem by using the same thinking that created it.
— ALBERT EINSTEIN

Veganomics (vee-gan-om-icks)—the art and science of rethinking everything we know about health, aging, weight loss, disease prevention and the footprint we leave on the world. My crazy vegan thing has colored everything in my life for the past twenty-five years. Most people find it militant and radical. It is. But it's so much fun, such a great way to live and be in the world. It means living consciously, compassionately, peacefully, at a healthy weight, with vitality and grace, in harmony with our environment, at peace with who we are and what we do.

The term *veganomics* was inspired by the bestselling book *Freakonomics* by Steven D. Levitt and Stephen J. Dubner, in which they examined the "hidden side of everything," from an economist's viewpoint. It was a totally new way of looking at how our society and our psyches operate. It questions the conventional explanations and puts a whole new spin on how we think about everything. I love that idea. To think veganomically I am asking that you rethink the way that you look at health, diet, disease and aging from a vegan perspective in order to create a whole new way of being in the world. This is my theory of relativity: What we choose to eat and the life-style choices we make are completely relative to who we are.

Nothing short of a total rethinking of what you know will change your current habits and your current state of health. And given all the marketing and brainwashing we face every hour of every day, that is no easy task.

Not an evening goes by that I am not ranting at the television screen, fuming over some pharmaceutical ad promising us freedom from disease and discomfort, while the breathy voice reading the disclaimer tells us the possible side effects. Frankly, they often sound a lot worse to me than the ailment's symptoms. Why is no one asking these pharmaceutical companies to make safer drugs for us? Why are we willing to accept drugs with side effects that will make us sick, but in a different way? And then they just offer us another drug to offset the damage of the current drug. We always seem to be on the hunt for the magic bullet—taking the easiest path, even though that path may lead nowhere that you'd want to go. That thinking has to change for us to be a healthy nation, because the way we live now is a recipe for a national disaster much worse than anything global warming or terrorists can throw our way.

Veganomics: From the Beginning

Who and what are vegetarians and vegans and where did this thinking come from? How did this thinking that has evolved into the veganism of today begin? What made people eschew meat and other animal food in the first place?

The first evidence of a vegetarian community shows up in Egypt, circa 3200 BC, when a vegetarian way of eating was adopted because of belief in the spiritual impact on one's reincarnation of eating blood. And it wasn't good. Eating blood held you back from evolution in your next life, inhibiting you from reaching nirvana and final peace.

Some anthropologists believe that vegetarianism dates back to before recorded history, and cites the digestive system of man as a piece of their evidence. Our digestive systems, it turns out, resembles those of herbivores far more than carnivores. No other meat-eating animal has molar teeth—only plant eaters and, well, humans. Anthropologists also cite as evidence the fact that humans contract so many life-threatening illnesses as a result of meat eating. Evolutionarily speaking, we are not built for it.

They further cite that while man obviously began to eat meat early on, it was not in quantities large enough to cause the species to evolve to accommodate such foods. It's believed to be the reason that feeding humans saturated fat can cause a spike in cholesterol, but feeding that same fat to a carnivorous animal has no impact on their cholesterol or on their health at all. Hmm…makes you think…

Vegetarians were at one time called Pythagoreans, named for the philosopher Pythagoras, who is said to have created the first organized vegetarian community in ancient Greece. This style of living and eating has waxed and waned in popularity for centuries. Throughout history, influential philosophers, world leaders and radical activists adopted a vegetarian lifestyle as a commentary on society, a spiritual practice, or an esoteric principle. From Leonardo da Vinci to Mohandas Gandhi, Leo Tolstoy to Martin Luther, Ben Franklin to Albert Einstein, vegetarians have very often been catalysts of change in their culture as well as advocates of compassion and equality.

But it wasn't until the mid-1800s that the term *vegetarianism* was actually coined by the British Vegetarian Society as a way to describe a lifestyle that was considered by them to be the key to a long and healthy life. The term *vegan* sprang from this same well about fifty years ago, when some members of the society decided that they didn't want to eat any kind of animal food whatsoever, including dairy products. Although veganism had been around for thousands of years (mostly practiced by religious sects), this was the first time it was named and organized as an offshoot of vegetarianism.

Vegetarianism is, and always has been, a voluntary way to live. Never in history was it forced on any group or community. Choosing to eschew animal food was most often accompanied by a specific ideology, which often comprised unconventional lifestyle choices such as an inclination toward pacifism and a desire to rebel against the standards of the day.

Veganomics: Growing Pains

Humans will naturally eat anything necessary for survival. Some think it's this ability to consume anything that led to our dominance over other species. Being able to adjust to varying climates, the exploration of new habitats, migration and the will to try new and alien foods are uniquely human characteristics. Animals, in most cases, are biologically dependent on certain climates and particular foods for survival. We definitely have an evolutionary advantage in the food department. We can survive anywhere and on almost anything—at least so far.

So vegetarianism or veganism was often the way to distinguish a community as well as make a social statement. Interestingly, the voluntary abstinence from foods can only be sustained by a well-fed community, where people have the time to reflect on the human condition and comment on society. Usually individualists and strongly opinionated, vegetarians have gained the reputation of being sharply critical of their culture. This observation holds true to this day.

Understanding the choice of early vegetarianism and how it differentiated a group of people can only come with the comprehension of the central role meat played in society. A sign of affluence and social standing, meat became a status symbol. The richer you were, the more meat you ate. With royalty and aristocracy often offering the common people little more than crushing oppression, there is no wonder that meat eating was equated with corruption and greed. Talk about you are what you eat!

Veganomics: America

As society continued to evolve and periods of affluence came and went influencing human eating patterns, vegetarian and vegan eating grew to be associated with social change and compassion. While always part of the landscape, vegetarian eating never enjoyed widespread enthusiasm, with veganism off in the hinterlands of the seriously radical minority. Health was not much of a factor and vegetarianism was not much more than a blip on the screen of the New World for the longest time. But vegetarianism wasn't really needed until the advent of the Industrial Revolution.

Until the mid-1900s, not much meat was eaten in America. The cost was sky-high; refrigeration was not widely available and distribution was problematic, at best. However, one of the "side effects" of our great Industrial Revolution was that meat grew relatively cheaper, because farmers were learning how to mass-produce it; it was easier to store because we had refrigeration and it was easier to distribute by rail and truck. Still, eating meat was a symbol of status and its consumption grew and grew with affluence—as did the incidence of heart disease, obesity, cancer and diabetes.

The social upheaval of the 1960s changed everything. Our youth revolted against the established ways of society, against the fact that it was, in their opinion, destroying the world. (Not far off base, as it turns out…) Choosing vegetarian and vegan eating habits that were radically different than their parents was just another way to revolt, along with the embracing of pacifism and protest of the Vietnam War. Out of this revolt, came what we now refer to as the "counterculture," a rejection of anything to do with the ruling "Establishment," the older generation that was bankrupting society—financially, spiritually, emotionally and physically. This revolution transcended class and culture, with great stress on ancient Eastern wisdom and a return to the land. A consciousness was born that could not be ignored or turned away from.

But it wasn't until 1971 that vegetarianism stepped out of the shadows and into the light of mainstream consciousness with the publication of Frances Moore Lappé's *Diet for a Small Planet*. As Lappé delved into issues of world hunger, she was stunned to discover that it takes fourteen times as much grain to feed an animal than what you get out of it in meat. The discovery of this terrible waste of resources drove her to write the defining manifesto of the early American vegetarian movement. Lappé's information is still (unfortunately) pertinent today, like the fact that livestock eat 80% of the grain grown in the United States and if each American cut his meat consumption by just 10%, there would be enough grain to feed every starving person in the world. Think about that. Reducing the amount of meat you consume by only 10% could literally change the world. That's about one meatless meal a week!

Diet for a Small Planet was a hit. And that was odd, since nothing could have been considered more weird than not eating meat in America in the 1970s. It was widely held that a person would starve or become seriously ill without meat, so Lappé prepared to address that criticism with her theory of protein combining or complementing, a now-debunked theory that plagues vegetarians—and especially vegans—to this day. In an attempt to convince readers they could get proper nutrients without meat, Lappé found and cited some studies done on rats that showed a particular amino acid combination that would provide nutrition similar to eating meat by specific combinations of whole grains and beans. The problem was and is that this was just a theory, with no studies ever conducted with humans. No one, even Lappé, considered that cows, pigs and chickens ate only grains and plants and were just fine on the protein front. Not one other herbivore worried about protein combining to be properly nourished. As valuable as her work was in shedding light on the waste of resources needed to produce meat, Lappé gave critics of vegetarian eating just the ammunition they needed to poke holes in the universal value of a plant-based diet, and in the process, created the stigma of malnourishment associated with vegetarian eating.

Just an aside…in 1981, with the reissue of her classic book, Lappé recanted her own theory with the truth: that if people eschewing meat are getting enough varied nutrients and eating whole grains, beans, vegetables, nuts and seeds, there is no problem with protein. But the debunked protein-combining theory persists even today.

Veganomics and Modern Health

With the light that *Diet for a Small Planet* shed on the production and consumption of meat in the twentieth century, there was no turning back for the vegetarian movement in this country. Out of this new awareness sprang the first vegetarian cookbooks, restaurants, food co-ops and communes, all dedicated to making a lighter footprint on the planet, safeguarding our animals and preserving human health.

In 1975, Australian ethics professor Peter Singer wrote *Animal Liberation*, the first academic work to present ethical arguments for not eating animals and not using them in lab experiments. A new fire was lit under the vegetarian movement. Seemingly overnight, animal rights groups cropped up all over the world and a new level of awareness was born.

By the 1980s the vegetarian movement was clicking along, enjoying life just outside the mainstream of American consciousness. Most people were still put off by the myth that vegetarianism required careful planning and could socially isolate one from friends and family.

But the biggest myths of all vegetarianism still persist. Many vegetarians believe that dairy and eggs are not only healthy but vital. Twenty years ago, not many people in and out of the movement in the United States had been thinking of life totally free from animal foods. The health consequences of dairy and eggs had not yet been widely published. And while *Diet for a Small Planet* was revered as the manifesto of vegetarianism, there was much more to be exposed about things like "factory farming" and the serious consequences of meat production on our health and environment.

In 1987, John Robbins published *Diet for a New America*. The heir to the Baskin-Robbins ice cream empire, Robbins walked away from his heritage and committed to a life of natural living, abandoning his world of privilege to live on a small island off British Columbia in a one-room cabin with his wife, where they grew most of their own food and lived off the land. During his ten years of self-imposed exile, Robbins realized the impact food production has on the planet and the effect of food consumption on human health. He wanted to things to change.

Robbins brought together all the information published on animal food production, health and the environment and distilled it into a powerful statement about eating animal food. *Diet for a New America* was not only exhaustively documented but was also unflinching in its graphic portrayal of the horrors of factory farming, the filth that surrounds meat production and the care and compassion lacking in commercial meat production.

Robbins painstakingly demonstrated how deadly meat-based diets are and how safe, healthy, balanced and environmentally wise it is to eat a vegan diet. And in the final chapters, he introduced the world to the terrible environmental consequences of animal agriculture. A long-time vegan himself, Robbins is largely responsible for helping to make "vegan" a widely recognized term.

But that's not all. In the five years immediately following the publication of *Diet for a New America*, meat consumption in the United States dropped 20%! His public relations campaign was aggressive with full-page ads in the *New York Times* and other major newspapers around the country. Featuring a fierce-looking Tyrannosaurus rex and the headline "How to Win an Argument with a Meat Eater," this brilliant ad was a laundry list of the damage done to our health and environment by meat production.

The ad still runs in an updated form on www.vegsource.com. Here's a small sampling of the statistics that will really help to change your thinking:

Number of people who could be adequately fed if Americans reduced their meat intake by 10%: 100 million

Pounds of potatoes grown on an acre: 40,000

Pounds of beef produced on an acre: 250

Percentage of U.S. farmland devoted to beef production: 56%

Pounds of grain and soybeans required to produce one pound of beef: 16

Percentage of corn grown in the United States eaten by livestock: 80%

Percentage of oats grown in the United States eaten by livestock: 95%

Number of acres of U.S forest cleared for cropland to produce a meat-based diet: 260 million

Increased risk of breast cancer for women who eat meat daily compared to once a week: 3.8 times

Increased risk of fatal prostate cancer for men who consume meat, dairy, eggs and milk daily: 3.6 times

Average risk of heart attack for a man who eats meat regularly: 50%

Average risk of heart attack for a man who doesn't eat meat: 15%

Number of medical schools in the United States: 125

Number that requires nutrition study: 30

Gallons of water to produce one pound of California beef: 5,000

Calories of fossil fuel expended to create 1 calorie of protein from beef: 78

Number of animals killed for meat per hour in the United States: 660,000

All these statistics are disturbingly true, and they prompted the scientific community and medical profession to sit up and take notice. That was good.

By the 1990s, medical evidence about the link between diet and health was becoming commonplace, with Dr. John McDougall being among the first to publish a series of books promoting a vegan diet as the way to prevent and even treat major illnesses. At around the same time, Dr. Dean Ornish rose to popularity with his program to reverse heart disease through a vegan diet. Organizations such as the American Dietetic Association, the American Cancer Society and the American Heart Association all published endorsements of vegetarian diets. Joining the powerful voices for change, Dr. Neal Barnard, president and founder of Physicians' Committee for Responsible Medicine, and Dr. T. Colin Campbell, author of *The China Study*, have taken up the standard and have become, with Drs. Ornish and McDougall, the voices of reason in the scientific community.

I knew vegetarianism had truly arrived when our own government finally abandoned the antiquated meat and dairy industry–sponsored "Four Food Groups" and replaced it with the new "Food Pyramid," which clearly shows that Americans should be eating a diet that consists largely of whole grains, vegetables, beans, fruits, nuts, seeds and good-quality fats. From my view, all we need to do is lop off the top of the pyramid, removing the meat, eggs and dairy—and it would be perfect.

The vegan movement continues to grow and evolve as the flower children of the sixties have turned into the graying baby boomers of today, with eating whole, unprocessed foods becoming the path to health, fitness and the preservation of youth. This generation has taken eating well to a new level, making it not only socially conscious, but very hip—yet, interestingly still a rebellion—only this time against the established thinking about health, disease, aging, medicine and the environment. Baby boomers are leading the revolution in questioning the conventional wisdom of how we prevent and treat illness. Alternative medicine, diets and lifestyles have stepped into the light of mainstream America because of the demand of this generation for a better and saner way to live and age.

As a vegan since 1983, I can tell you that this is a welcome change for me. I often say that once people experience a life of true health—one that can only be discovered through eating real food—they can't imagine how well a human can feel. With adopting a vegan approach to eating comes an acute sense of being awake. I often likened this new awareness to having a veil lifted off my eyes. Clarity of thought, focus, serenity, strength of mind and body must be experienced. It is our birthright to feel well, strong and vital.

George Bernard Shaw said it best: "The odd thing about being a vegetarian is not that the things that happen to other people do not happen to me—they all do—but they happen differently: pain is different, pleasure different, fever different, cold different; even love is different."

VEGANOMICS: THE CHALLENGE

But before getting all warm and cozy and comfy in the growth of the vegan movement, let's be aware of the something of a backlash in the past few years. Maybe we got tired of every expert that could read at the third-grade level telling us what to eat and what was healthy. Maybe we got tired of all the conflicting information. Maybe we got tired of being lectured. See, vegans can be a real pain in the butt. I know; I am one and sometimes our passion can drive us to preach about compassion and kindness from high atop a soapbox. All that self-righteousness, spray painting fur coats and finger wagging can be a real turnoff. We can come off as high-minded and exclusionary, making people feel less than wonderful about themselves. You know I'm right.

But it would take more than a couple of Birkenstock-wearing militants to prompt the resurgence we have seen in meat eating. It's more likely that our very own meat industry lobby has something to do with it. This lobby strongly supported the passage of food disparagement laws that make it illegal to criticize perishable food products. Think about it; they even sued Oprah for saying that she'd think twice before she had another burger.

Meanwhile, the debate about animal products, chemicals, organics, production and the environment will continue to rage. The fight will be played out on the evening news and in the courts of America. It will also be fought by the consumer, with their dollars in supermarkets, and in their kitchens. It is important to sift through all the spin and see who profits from the information you see. My rule of thumb is that if the beneficiary is some multinational corporation, I question what I read or hear. If the beneficiary is humanity or the planet, I am all in.

VEGANOMICS AND YOU

I think that everyone is in their own spot in their evolution and I don't think that vegetarians or vegans are necessarily better people. We just see things differently and our footprint on the planet can be lighter than others. I don't consider my fellow humans to be children who need to be scolded about their choices, but I believe that all people when presented with the best option for great health will take the right path, to their best ability. I am concerned about people's health, the planet's health and the future we will leave to our children. The fact that compassionate living comes with it is a wonderful side benefit that I love about this lifestyle.

And the facts support my passion. Our collective health is in serious decline and I think that only a radical approach to eating (and for our meat-eating culture, trust me: this is radical) will save that collective health. Just as we all believe that radical societal change is the only thing that will preserve what is left of the environment, so it goes with our health. In fact, the most inconvenient truth is that animal food—the world's largest single source of pollution—is also the world's single-largest contributor to degenerative disease. With 2,500 Americans dying each and every day from some form of cardiovascular disease, most of which can be directly linked to the consumption of saturated fats, it's time to take notice.

Is It All or Nothing?

While some vegans may disagree with me, I think there are levels of commitment when it comes to vegan living and the more you live this lifestyle, the more you will evolve and change. You may find that your commitment to living a vegan life goes way beyond fitting into a single-digit-size pair of jeans or having a smaller gut. You may find that your crazy vegan life makes you a healthier person, a more conscious citizen who leaves a lighter footprint on the planet and influences the way people eat and the way we treat animals.

Life is so much bigger than the perimeter of our plates, but that is where many of us are stuck. We are so trapped in our food choices that we are missing what the world has to offer. Our obsession with eating has left us spiritually and emotionally bankrupt as we stuff our mouths with food that is pure trash. We blame it on the stress of our overscheduled lives. We say that we are overwhelmed and need junk food, fast food, meat, milk, ice cream, sugar, candy, cookies and cheese for comfort and familiarity in an uncomfortable world. We need to sink onto the couch and "veg out" (strange term for lethargy…) to de-stress.

Look, everyone needs help at some point or another. I surely did and sometimes still do. I am just saying that we should be inspired by all that we see and hear to think for ourselves; to create change; shake up our lives. I wrote this book to inspire you to rethink and change your life, your health, your body and your destiny. Our modern world can easily turn us into non-thinking zombies. Take your life back and create the one you want.

One Step at a Time

As for what and how much to change, vegetarianism is a seemingly endless continuum. You may decide to begin slowly, giving up just meat, and then refine your food choices as you evolve and see results, eventually eliminating all animal food from your diet. Then you'll really see results. It is the rare person who goes "cold turkey" from standard American fare to pure, organic vegan eating. Most of us, myself included, started by getting rid of meat and chicken. Personally, I hung on to dairy foods for a good number of years and then dumped milk, cheese, eggs, yogurt and ice cream twenty-five years ago. I have never looked back. I have never felt better.

But take care. Don't just give up meat, eggs and chicken and subsist on sugar and junk food just because they are "vegan." Junk is junk and it will make you sick and fat, whether vegan or not, organic or not. When Leonardo da Vinci, Gandhi and Albert Einstein decided they would adopt a vegetarian lifestyle as a commentary on their societies and out of love and respect for animals and all living things, you can rest assured they didn't replace meat with Snickers and Coke.

A few years ago, I was reading a vegetarian cooking magazine and I was enraged at the amount of sugar, white flour and other compromised ingredients that were being used in the recipes. Sure, it was all vegan, but yikes! I was ranting to a friend who said, "The magazine is vegan; that doesn't always mean healthy." She was right. If you fall into that trap, you'll feel just as crappy as you do now.

Go vegan in a healthy way and you will be loving life.

Top Ten Reasons to Go Vegan

If all of this hasn't convinced you, here are my reasons to go vegan. I think these will do the trick. If not, I have to say that I don't really know what will make you stop killing yourself with an unhealthy diet and start living a whole, healthy, fit life.

Eating a vegan diet and living a natural lifestyle will be the best decisions of your life. There is more than enough scientific research that clearly demonstrates the health benefits of a plant-based diet for both us and the planet.

1. You can prevent disease. A plant-based diet is way healthier than the Standard American Diet and is the best at preventing, treating and even reversing heart disease, diabetes and high blood pressure. A vegan diet has been proven to reduce the risk of many cancers and even alleviate many of the symptoms that go along with that dreaded disease. And you avoid most, if not all of the obesity-related illnesses we suffer with, because eating vegan is the best way to lose excess weight safely and keep it off. (See #2.)

Science has shown that the single most effective way to stop the literal onslaught of coronary heart disease or to prevent it completely is to eat a natural, whole vegetarian diet. Look, heart attacks and cardiovascular disease kill more than 1 million men and women every single year and hold the dubious crowns of being the leading causes of death in this fine country of ours. But according to Joel Furman, MD, author of *Eat to Live*, the mortality rate for cardiovascular disease (the risk drops to 15%) is lower among vegetarians because they naturally consume no animal fat and less cholesterol, but do eat more fiber and antioxidant-rich vegetables and fruit, creating a base of health that is off the charts.

It doesn't take a rocket scientist to figure out that eating meat and dairy is a horror show for your health. You'll look and feel tired and wiped out. You'll be fat and bloated. You're likelier to die younger. Life will suck because you never feel well.

2. You will lose weight and keep it off. The way that most Americans eat—lots of saturated fats, processed foods, sugar and chemicals and very few vegetables, fruits, whole grains and other nutrient-rich foods is making us fat, fat, fat.

According to the Centers for Disease Control and Prevention, 65% of adults and 17% of our young children (ages six to nineteen) are overweight or obese, increasing their risks of heart disease, diabetes, stroke and cancer. The latest research shows us that, if we don't put an end to this madness, this is the first time in history that life expectancy will be reduced because there is too much to eat, instead of too little.

Dean Ornish, MD, president of the Preventive Medicine Research Institute in California, found that overweight people who adopted a plant-based diet lost an average of twenty-four pounds in the first year just by giving up animal foods and had kept that weight off more than five years later. Do you know of any other diets that can tout those kinds of statistics? And did I mention that they did it without obsessive measuring, counting calories, skipping carbs or feeling hungry, deprived and cranky?

3. You will live a longer and healthier life. Michael Roizen, MD, author of *The RealAge Diet*, says that rethinking your food choices and eating a vegetarian diet can add about thirteen healthy years to your life. He adds that people who eat most of their calories from animal food, loaded with saturated fats and excessive calories, live shorter lives and experience more physical and mental disabilities and sexual dysfunction in their time on this planet. Animal foods also clog arteries, steal your vitality and inhibit your immune function.

And if you think this is just the ranting of a broccoli-crazed vegan, think again. Residents of Okinawa, Japan, experience the longest life expectancy and the most robust health of anyone in the world. According to a thirty-year study of more than six hundred Okinawan centenarians, their diet of unrefined complex carbohydrates, like brown rice, fiber-rich vegetables, fruit and soy foods are the keys to health and vitality. We would be wise to mimic their way of life.

4. You will have stronger, healthier bones. This one is easy; just connect the following dots. Animal protein is best digested by serum calcium in your blood. When there isn't enough calcium in the bloodstream, your body leaches it from your bones. The result is that over time our calcium-deprived skeletons become porous and weak as more and more calcium is used to digest animal protein.

Most experts agree that the best way to keep your bones healthy is to get the calcium you need from your food (with supplementation used as your condition requires), just the way nature intended. The good news is that the right foods automatically also supply you with the nutrients needed to support your use of calcium, vitamin D, phosphorus and magnesium.

But before you pick up that glass of milk, think about this: You can get all the calcium you need from beans, tofu, tempeh and leafy greens like collards, kale, turnip greens and broccoli. And this calcium is readily available to your bones without the side effects of milk, which can include lactose intolerance, bloating, gas, diarrhea, growth hormones, pesticides and herbicides (in commercial dairy), allergies, obesity, sinus congestion and even increased risks of some cancers.

5. You'll have lots more energy. Eat your vegetables and skip the meat, the chips, the candy, the soda, and all the other junk. Good nutrition gives your body fuel it can use, so you have more energy for your daily adventures. Balanced vegetarian diets are free of artery-clogging fats and cholesterol, which deprive your muscles of essential oxygen and make you sluggish and lethargic. Because whole grains, vegetables, beans, fruit, nuts and seeds are so amazingly rich in complex carbohydrates, vitamins, minerals and other essential nutrients they give you plenty of the best high-octane fuel that your body needs to function like the finely crafted machine it is.

6. You'll be a part of the solution to pollution, not part of the problem. Once you realize the devastation that the meat industry is having on our planet, you will run to the closest produce section and stock up…and walk right past the meat case. Veggies are good for you, good for the planet and good for your conscience. According to the Environmental Protection Agency, chemical and animal waste runoff from factory farms is responsible for more than 173,000 miles of polluted rivers and streams. It has been predicted that farmland runoff will become one of the greatest threats to our water quality. Some of the biggest offenders include confined animal facilities, pesticides in feed and manure, pesticide spraying, irrigation and fertilizing. (See chapter 3.)

7. You can help wipe out world hunger and end cruelty to animals. About 80% of all the grain products produced in the United States go to feed livestock. The billions of livestock animals in the United States eat more than five times the grain that Americans themselves eat. Studies at Cornell University show that if all the grain being fed to animals was fed to people instead, we would have food for almost 800 million hungry mouths. And if we exported some of that grain to other countries in need of food, we could boost U.S. exports by $80 billion a year!

According to www.goveg.com, some 7 to 10 billion animals are slaughtered each year for human dining in the United States alone. But unlike the cows, pigs and chickens that lived on the mythical "Old MacDonald" farm of children's rhymes, most animals today are factory farmed, crammed into tight spaces where they can barely move. They are fed diets that are tainted with pesticides, growth hormones (so we can get our burgers faster) and antibiotics (because they are forced to live so unnaturally that they grow sick more easily). These pathetic creatures are not protected by any laws either; in fact, most farm animals are exempt from state anticruelty laws.

Gandhi once said that you could judge the quality of a culture by the way they treat their animals. Think about that.

8. You'll save money. The price of a steak is far greater than a head of broccoli. The cost of meat accounts for more than 10% of the average

American food budget, beaten only by eating out and junk food. On average, Americans eat two hundred pounds of chicken, meat and fish each year. Eating whole grains, vegetables, beans, soy, fruits, nuts and seeds can save you about $4,000 dollars in food costs annually—and thousands in health-care costs as time goes by, since you will be less likely to become one of the statistics that is causing our health-care costs to spiral out of control.

9. Your dinner plate will be a work of art. Monet would be envious of the color that decorates your dining table. It's the disease-battling antioxidants and phytochemicals that give vegetables and fruit their stunning hues. Those rich colors not only treat our eyes, but tell us that the food we are eating is rich in anthocyanins and carotenoids.

Yellow and orange veggies like carrots, sweet potatoes, mangoes, pumpkin, corn and butternut squash get their brilliant color from carotenoids; leafy greens owe their vibrant color to chlorophyll; red, blue and purple foods like plums, cherries, blueberries, beets, red bell peppers, blackberries, red cabbage and raspberries are rich sources of anthocyanins. If you can cook and "eat by color" you'll ensure that you get all the immune-boosting, disease-preventing nutrients that nature has to offer us.

10. It's so easy. I would never lie to you. Honestly, if you can find your way to the kitchen and read above the first-grade level, you can prepare a great vegan dinner. With all the tastes, textures and nutrients that nature has given you, you will never be bored or lack inspiration.

And yes, I want you to cook from scratch as much as possible. Seven days a week would be just great but if you need some help at the end of a particularly long, busy day, you need look no further than your local supermarket's freezer section. With all the vegan options available now, from pot pies to pizza to side dishes, there is really no excuse not to eat well. Just read the labels carefully and avoid any additives you don't want to eat and watch the sodium levels. Restaurants and casual dining joints, even street lunch carts are all getting on the bandwagon and realizing that we veggie types are here to stay—and we want food that is delicious, satisfying, varied and truly healthy for us. So you get to benefit from all that newfound awareness!

Vegan Myths I Love

MYTH: *A vegan diet lacks essential nutrients like protein, calcium and iron.*
TRUTH: You may assume that protein and iron must come from meat and calcium from dairy products; the truth is that whole grains, beans, nuts, seeds and vegetables will provide us with all the protein we need. Broccoli has more protein, ounce for ounce, than any meat. Iron can come in many veggie forms, including dark leafy greens, lentils and other beans. For calcium, look to dark leafy greens, almonds, sesame seeds, black beans and sea veggies.

MYTH: *You must be a rocket scientist to make all the proper nutrient combinations to be healthy on a vegan eating plan.*
TRUTH: Old thinking said that vegetarians could not get proper protein in a balanced form because certain amino acids are missing that make the protein more useable in the body. No special combining is needed to be certain that you are getting what you need. You just need eat a wide variety of foods—whole grains, veggies, beans. All other vitamins and nutrients are as readily available in a vegan diet as they are in an animal food diet, without the side effects.

However, there is no reliable source of vitamin B_{12} in a vegan diet. While there are fortified food choices, supplementation is the best way to get this essential vitamin. New vegans are not at risk because stores of B_{12} will last for three to five years at the very least. A simple blood test will reveal whether or not supplementation is needed.

MYTH: *Eating meat is traditional and natural for humans.*
TRUTH: Many of history's worst abominations have hidden behind the

excuse of "tradition," so you can skip that one. As for the "naturalness" of eating meat, well, technically, humans are omnivores, meaning that we can eat just about anything. If you look at the structure of the human anatomy, you will see that we have a small percentage of tearing teeth, designed for meat eating. The majority of our teeth are grinders, for grains and vegetables. Our digestive tract also differs from carnivores. The long, convoluted tubes that make up our intestines hold on to bacteria from meat, wreaking havoc internally, causing poor digestion, body odor and failing health.

MYTH: *Vegans have a hard time eating out.*
TRUTH: I always say that I can eat anywhere and it's true. From steakhouses to international cafes to neighborhood joints on the corner, restaurants have gotten the message that vegetarians are here to stay and that we want more to eat than a baked potato and artfully arranged snow peas when we dine out. There is always something that I can find to satisfy my tastes without getting on a soapbox in front of the waitstaff and without asking them to create a new dish that doesn't appear on the menu.

MYTH: *It's too expensive to eat a vegan diet.*
TRUTH: A pound of veal costs $7.99–$8.99. A pound of tofu is $1.49. A pound of carrots is $.89. Any more questions? Of course, if you are feeding your family on the special 99-cent menu at the Golden Arches, then I can't compete. But your eventual health-care costs will far outpace my personal preferences for expensive olive oil.

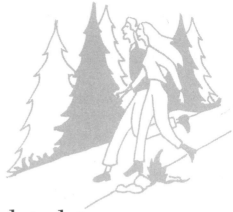

3

The Path to Rethinking Your Life

Whether industrialized societies can cure themselves of their meat addictions may ultimately be a greater factor in world health than all the doctors, health insurance policies and drugs put together.

—THE CHINA-OXFORD-CORNELL PROJECT ON NUTRITION

I bet you thought I would leave twisting in the wind with a bunch of menus, recipes and exercises as your only tools (although we have those, too) to help you make significant changes in your life. If I wanted you to fail, I would write yet another in the seemingly endless line of books telling you that if you tweak this and substitute that, exercise five minutes a day and take a few supplements, you will have the slim, leanly muscled supermodel body you crave. That would be too easy, too much of the same stuff that made us fatter, the world messier, our kids unhealthier and the self-help gurus richer.

I want so much for you. I know that sounds noble and you may be wondering why I care. Sure, I make money in my work; this book isn't free. But my mission is to show you that you can have health, fitness, your ideal weight and leave the planet a better place for your presence here. You can avoid the illnesses that come from a sedentary life.

Vegan living means a big life change for most people. For it to work fully for you, you must first commit. Yes, there's that *C* word! And there are five basic principles on this path to your new life that are essential to your success, if you are to live the life you were meant to have:

- Prepare
- Make Choices
- Eat Well
- Get Moving
- Reconnect

Embracing these principles may not be as hard as you imagine, but it's not as easy as some may have you believe. Once you understand and engage the power of each of these concepts and make them the foundation of your life, you will be blown away by what you can achieve.

Prepare

Now is the time to decide who you want to be in this world. Now is the time to prepare to change your life, to rethink everything you thought you knew about weight loss and health.

Lasting weight loss and enduring health are not just about your body. This is the principle that will help you engage your head and your heart. You will take an honest look at your life and what you want. This is the point at which you finally accept the simple truths of weight loss—eat less, eat real food, exercise more. Prepare to live fully and vitally, to eat delicious and satisfying food that you have prepared lovingly and mindfully—without sacrificing a single living creature in that process. Prepare to live a life without deprivation and without neurotic, obsessive guilt!

Your journey to good health starts with a conscious *intention* to live in a new way. What do you want from this life change? Do you simply want to be slimmer? Do you want to plant a garden, free of arthritic pain? Do you want to have the strength to lift your children or grandchildren onto your shoulders? Do you want to recapture some of your youthful vitality and strength? Do you want to change your life so that you can live with more energy and joy? Do you want to alleviate, eliminate or prevent an acute or chronic health condition? Do you want to live compassionately and stop contributing to cruelty? Do you want to leave the world a better place?

Whatever your intention, don't limit yourself with thinking about the numbers on the scale or on your clothing label…or by the size of your dream. If you want it, whatever "it" is, you will attract…or repel it with your thinking. If you view a life change as hard and challenging, it will be hard and challenging. If you think that this will be yet another diet that fails, then unfortunately, you will fail. If you see it as an exciting new adventure, that's exactly what you will get.

Positive Changes Begin with Positive Thinking

Positive thinking can change everything for you. But positive thinking is not so easy to achieve and maintain. We live in a culture that sets us up for failure and cashes in on our insecurities. Every television ad we see is telling us that we are losers, but if we buy their pills, perfume, lotion, burger, drink, mouthwash, clothes or car, we will be sane, sexy, smart, funny, healthy, fit and thin. These messages reinforce the notion that we cannot be good enough or healthy enough without their products, that what they are selling will make us whole, complete humans.

But for your own survival, you must *change the way you think*. In the *Tao Te Ching*, Lao Tzu says that if a man cannot change his thoughts, then he will not change anything. Without changing your thinking or with resistance to that change, you will fail. *Seriously, you will fail.* And you will add this book to the pile of others that didn't work for you. And you'll go on thinking that nothing can help you. But the truth is simple: Only *you* can help you—with a little guidance and support from me. And it all starts in your head.

I'm saying rethink everything—and then change what you need to. But change is hard, especially when it comes to breaking a lifetime of bad habits.

Habits form in the brain. (I told you, it all starts in your head.) When we do something repetitively, our brains and bodies go in to autopilot, functioning without much thought. Mindless eating and unconscious living means we eat too much—and too much of all the wrong things, exercise too little, depend on pharmaceuticals to keep us up and keep us down.

We get into a rut. Our life becomes routine, replete with habits that are not contributing to our health and wellness, so we have to give ourselves a good shaking up or we'll continue in this downward spiral that is typical of our culture of indulgence and convenience.

Replace Old Habits with Conscious Living

Letting old habits fade and new ones take their place starts with developing a positive vision of the outcome you want. Too often, dwelling on the negative—your current state of health—overwhelms your efforts to change. When you focus on how much you hate being overweight or what a drag it is to be tired all the time, it is impossible to make room for the positive emotions that will carry you to your goals. It's really simple. If you think that you can't do something, then you probably can't do it. (In high school I was on the swim team and I was having a tough time keeping up with the hard, fast interval drills. The coach yelled down to me, "Stop telling yourself that you can't do this!" And when I did that, I swam like never before.) To move forward, you've got to ask yourself what your life will be like as you change. How will your life be enhanced? What will the benefits be for you, your family, your community and your world? If you have a clear vision of how your life will be different, you can bring that vision into being. Your mind is a powerful tool.

New habits, healthy habits can be created by reprogramming yourself and taking your brain off autopilot for a while. The key to lasting weight loss and health is to simply reinforce a new practice. But here is the cool thing: Whatever actions you take—and repeat—will become automatic in a mere twenty-one days. Just as your present lifestyle may be killing you now, it can quickly be turned around to become your source of strength, health and fitness. Take a walk after dinner, replace a high-fat, sugar-laden muffin with a healthier breakfast choice, skip that after-work beer for a half hour at the gym. Simple actions that you start now will become habits that will reap immeasurable benefits: You'll sleep better; have fewer mood swings; lose weight; get toned; develop stamina; have gorgeous skin and hair; and age naturally and gracefully in a strong, healthy body free of the aches, pains and chronic annoyances that plague our modern world.

Sure, one day we will all die and become compost, but aren't you entitled to live well in health and happiness while you are here?

Make Choices

It's one thing to have your head in the game, feeling like you are ready to make real change for tangible, lasting results. But it's the choices you make and the actions you take that will determine how much you change and how quickly you see the results you crave.

Every day we are faced with choices; but too many of us ignore them and opt for what's habitual or "normal." Living your life on autopilot— unconsciously doing things that will make you fat and unhealthy—is a choice. You can decide to engage positive thinking and replace bad habits with mindfulness.

Eating huge portions of meat and dairy products has become the norm. But since our bodies have actually evolved to thrive on a diet comprising 75 to 80% plants, with a very small percentage of animal foods, do we really need to choose foods that slow the metabolism or contribute substantially to obesity and heart disease? Eating meat is unnecessary. It sabotages our ability to lose weight and maintain that loss. And meat will kill us.

Making your food choices from the plant kingdom will have an enormous positive impact on everything: your body, your skin, your hair, your energy— even your attitude and emotions. Whole grains, vegetables, beans and bean products, fruits, nuts, seeds and healthy oils all work in the body to support organ function so that every day you can achieve your personal best.

If you are caught in the endless circle that takes you from bed to fridge to car to work to couch to fridge to bed, you can choose to break the cycle. Take a walk after dinner, hit the gym, park two blocks away from your office (or get off the bus a stop sooner), hide the remote…You can make a hundred little choices every day that will get your heart pumping and your muscles working.

When we walk instead of drive, select fresh organic produce instead of packaged and processed food, turn down the heat a couple of degrees, turn off the water tap, recycle, reuse and rethink, these choices will have an immediate and lasting impact on our bodies, our spirits and our planet.

EAT WELL

Of course, eating well is a major aspect of this process and you'll find lots of invaluable information in the chapters ahead, but there are three aspects of eating well that you will want to keep in mind as you read and start making changes in your own life: what to eat, how to eat and when to eat (or not).

What to Eat

I cannot stress enough the importance of choosing fresh, whole foods as the foundation of your diet. I often say that we are starving ourselves to obesity. As a society, we eat a tremendous quantity of food (or something that resembles food), but little of it is fresh and alive, so we are constantly seeking more. The goal is to feel sated and vitalized by our food, not depleted. Eating foods that are inappropriate for you triggers you to eat more because you are not getting what you need... and you grow fatter and sicker. It's time to get off the merry-go-round of meat, sugar and dairy and get on board with whole grains, beans, vegetables (lots and lots of them!), nuts, seeds and healthy fats. Then and only then will you see the changes in your body and health that you crave.

But one rule never changes: To lose weight you must use more calories than you take in. This really is the simplest and easiest to understand theory. Calories in, calories out! Sure, it's sometimes hard to actually do it, since we're bombarded by food 24/7. But isn't it time to grow up and be responsible? We are no longer like our ancient ancestors, never knowing when the next meal will come wandering by the campfire or concerned that we'll be beaten to the berry bushes by some aggressive bear. Ours is a society of abundance. By simply choosing to eat regularly and sensibly, your metabolism will be stoked and you are on your way. Remember the first principle: Prepare with positive thinking. Along with the nutritional information, meal plans and recipes that I provide in this book you will be well equipped to achieve success for a lifetime.

How to Eat

Your body is a creature of habit and it loves routine. It likes knowing that things will happen in an orderly and peaceful way. It is one of the reasons we respond so poorly to stress and lack of order. Our bodies can't cope with it. Chaos in any form, on any level, causes your body to have a very strong response, some kind of defensive move. It wants to protect itself.

People who eat regularly, sitting down for each meal and snack are more likely to be in control of what they eat and how much. They are also more likely to have control of their weight. It works like this. When your body is being fed at regular intervals, it is much more likely to give up any excess when you exercise, burning up stores rather than, well, storing. Your body knows that you will be feeding it again so there is no risk of starvation. But when your eating pattern is chaotic, the body becomes wary: Why are nutrients coming in so erratically? Are you starving me? Am I under attack? The response to this uncertainty is to slow the metabolism to prevent the loss of calories that you may need to survive. The more erratic your eating habits are, the less likely you are to achieve and maintain a normal weight. (There's more about this under the next section, "When to Eat".)

Look at the way you eat. Do you sit down calmly at the table, enjoying each bite? Do you stand over the sink gulping down food from a plastic container? Do you eat while driving, walking, talking on your cell phone, watching the news, at your desk, while on the Internet, fighting with your kids and spouse...in other words, in utter chaos? If meal- or snacktime is less than pleasureable for you, then you need to change the way you do it. Your body depends on you to nourish it with the best nutrients and under the best conditions. You've probably seen those ads for pills that help the body to regulate cortisol, the stress hormone that when out of balance leads to excess belly fat. Living under stress is bad enough, but eating under stress guarantees that you will struggle with your weight. Cortisol is important but you don't need a pill to regulate it. When you make the conscious choice to create a friendly, calm environment in which to eat the best foods, it makes a huge difference to cortisol production—and the general stress of your life.

And speaking of huge, you also need to give up the notion that you have to eat until you are "Thanksgiving full." For most of us, we are not fighting over every scrap on the table. Eat consciously, chewing each mouthful until it is liquefied, and put your fork down between each bite. This advice is not new—you've probably heard it from your mother a hundred times. Speed kills, on the highway and at the dinner table. And it's not just about etiquette. It's for the good of your health. By eating slowly and consciously, our brains are able to register "fullness" (scientists say it takes about twenty minutes) at the appropriate time and you will naturally stop eating before you feel stuffed. Wolfing down your food also denies you the sensual experience of food.

When to Eat

Deciding that you will eat at regular intervals is an important element to your success. By choosing—and sticking to—regular times for every meal and snack not only will you be better able to keep your caloric intake under control, your body will be better able to use those calories and they won't end up being stored as fat!

There is also a time when *not* to eat. When you are creating your eating schedule, subtract three hours from the time you go to bed. That is the hour at which you must stop eating—completely! No exceptions. Not one morsel. Not a grape, a chocolate chip or a crouton. Nothing, nada, niente. If you're really desperate, have a cup of hot, clear tea. By eating close to bedtime, your body has to work hard to digest this food, when, in fact, it should be resting, rejuvenating and recovering, renewing cells and allowing organs to rest as well. After a day of eating, and particularly if you have been active, the body will continue to burn calories you have eaten throughout the day. If you eat right up until bedtime, the body at rest will not be able to burn off the excess calories. Stop eating three hours before bed and your metabolism will gently continue to chug along, burning and not storing.

Not only does eating too close to bedtime inhibit weight loss, but if your body is working to digest food all night, you will wake up tired and cranky. Inevitably you will lose your inspiration and motivation if you are always tired. Studies show that people who are even a little sleep-deprived or tired are more likely to turn to junk food as solace.

And last, that little nighttime hunger pang is your body burning fat stores, so don't curse it; thank it for being such a brilliant machine. While we might think of going to bed hungry as a punishment—memories of childhood discipline come to mind—believe me, you won't starve. Once your head hits that pillow, you'll sleep better for not having given in to the urge, and you'll wake up in a much better frame of mind.

Begin your day with breakfast. Your mother probably preached this message and I am here to do the same. The first food of the day is a big part of weight loss success and overall health and vitality. Countless studies have shown that people who eat breakfast eat much less throughout the day. Here's why: When you wake up, your blood sugar is a little low because you have not eaten all night while you slept (see above). So you need to stoke your metabolism, balance your blood sugar but avoid shocking your system with bad food choices. (The fat- and sugar-filled muffins are out! Whole grain, fresh fruit and veggies—yes, veggies—are in. Check out my breakfast menus and recipes for some really incredible choices.)

By mid-morning, you will be ready for your snack, which you will wisely keep under one hundred calories of whole grains or some protein, like peanut or other nut butter.

Because your body has been well-nourished by a healthy breakfast and snack, it will be simmering along so you won't be absolutely starving. A well-balanced lunch comprised of protein, carbohydrates and veggies will keep you going.

As the afternoon wanes and your energy starts to flag, an afternoon energy booster—some complex carbohydrates and protein—will work the best for you.

Dinner, eaten at least three hours before you go to bed, should be satisfying and easy to digest. While the traditional approach is to have a "big" meal at the end of the day, you will want to strive to keep this one fairly light but satisfying. Eating a plant-based diet makes it a whole lot easier to do this rather than making your body cope with meat—even chicken—that is hard to digest. Plant-based proteins and vegetables are the best choices, with just a small amount of carbohydrate for energy. (See my menu suggestions in chapter 6.)

GET MOVING

I can hear the groans already. This is worse than the food, right? The thought of sweating and straining at the gym, surrounded by fit, trim Barbie dolls and G. I. Joes just makes your blood run cold. But I'm here to help you make your blood run hot! And I'm sorry (which is the only apology you'll hear from me on this topic), but exercise is absolutely essential to weight loss and a healthy life.

If exercise hasn't been a part of your life before, it is never too late to start. Like everything else I ask of you in this book, it starts with your intention to get healthy and fit and requires your commitment to see it through. You have to make it a habit, just like cleaning your teeth every day. (You wouldn't dream of telling your dentist that you didn't have time for daily dental hygiene and expect him to prescribe a pill to replace brushing and flossing.) Exercise has to become just that kind of priority in your life. No excuses. No nonsense.

But I know what you're thinking: I don't have the time to exercise. When it comes to your health, you have to think like a smart financial planner. Pay yourself first. You have to be fit to fulfill all those personal, family and community obligations that you're now using as excuses not to exercise. What good is it if you are too tired to play with the kids, too stressed to function at your best at work, too beaten down to fight off every passing cold or infection?

You've probably read many of those articles about how to fit fitness into your day: walk to the store, park farther away from your destination, take the stairs, walk around the perimeter of the soccer field while the kids practice. Well, I have a news flash for you: These things work! You will see results with every change you make. But you have to put your heart in it. If you take an after-dinner stroll, then your results will be much less obvious than if you walk briskly... or jog! And these results you see will motivate you to do more, learn more, work harder, and maybe even head to a gym.

You don't have to become a gym rat to achieve fitness, but it can be a lot more effective and more fun if you join a local club. Not only will you have access to good advice, you'll also be more motivated and inspired by everyone around you—trainers and members alike. You're all in this thing together, working toward the same goals. Whether you're naturally competitive or just want the structure that a gym can provide, you'll find what you need.

Look for a gym that's close to your home or office. Don't give yourself another excuse not to exercise. A half hour at lunch time can make all the difference—it'll energize you for the rest of the day and the rest of your life. Make it as easy as possible to get to it... and go!

But if you feel you're not ready for the gym, that's okay. I'm going to give you a great home workout that's fun and invigorating. (See chapter 7, "Get Moving.") When you're ready to get out into the world, you'll find you can take your fitness to a whole new level—and love it.

You have to rethink how you will spend your days but once you start including regular exercise in your routine, you'll never go back.

RECONNECT

For many of us, trouble began when we became disconnected from our own bodies. Think about it. You didn't go to bed last night healthy and fit only to wake up and, surprise, you are fat and unhealthy this morning. It took time for you to gain that weight, for your energy levels to flag, for your organs to stop doing their jobs, for your muscles to stop holding you up—and it will take time to get things running smoothly again. The good news is that your body *wants* to be strong and healthy, so it will respond to healthy habits quickly. A lifetime of unhealthy eating habits and lack of exercise can be turned around in mere weeks, if you put your mind to it and change the way you do things now.

To succeed, you first need to change the way you think about your body. I'm not talking about flirting with yourself in the mirror. I'm talking about thinking about your body, what it is and does. The first thing may be that you realize you haven't thought about it at all, except to notice how fat and bloated you are or how old and achy, but you think that's normal. The last time you thought about your body may have been when you asked a trusted friend "Does this make me look fat?" Guess what? If you have to ask that question, you already know the answer.

It is time to reconnect with your body, its needs and its power. This body that you abuse with too much food, too much soda, sugar, chemicals, too little exercise and too little care is such an amazing—and forgiving—home. You might laugh at the old hippie saying that your body is a temple, but it's true. Take a good, hard look at what you ask of your body each and every day and then think about what you do for it in return. You will most likely see that your body is getting the short end of the stick in this deal. Dr. Mehmet Oz said on an episode of *Oprah* that we should think about how we would treat someone else's body. We are unlikely to abuse someone else's, but consider what you are doing to your own.

It's time to wake up and commit to caring for your true home in this life. You change the oil in your car on a regular basis, clean the house, wash the clothes, mow the lawn, weed the garden. But your body? We take better care of our car engines than our organs and we wonder why we feel like we do.

Write It Down

Being conscious of the choices you make is the beginning. But how do you begin? Many people find that keeping a diary of what they eat keeps them honest and completely aware of what they are putting in their mouths. There is something powerful about writing it down, even though you will be the only person who sees the pages. You can't (or at least shouldn't) lie to yourself when you write it down in black and white. There is no more denial when what you eat is right there on the pages before you. Your diary is your personal record of where you've been and how you've progressed. And it is probably the best way to develop conscious eating habits that will serve you for the rest of your life.

A personal diary is equally valuable to keep track of whatever exercise program you choose to adopt. Even recording those baby steps—a walk around the block, playing catch in the backyard, getting off the bus a few blocks before your destination, taking the stairs instead of the elevator—will give you a sense of accomplishment and inspire you to do more and fill up those pages.

The following chapters will give you all the hints, tips, strategies and information you'll need for your journey to health. But you might find yourself coming back to this chapter as a reminder of the basic principles that are the core of this lifetime plan: prepare, make choices, eat well, get moving and reconnect.

Food for Thought

Knowledge is power. —SIR FRANCIS BACON

Reading this book may not be the first time you've taken steps to be healthier, get more fit or be "greener," but it's my hope that once you've read through to the final page—and started to put some of what you've learned into action—that you'll stop worrying about all this and learn to love life and yourself again. It's time to get it together so you can get on with it.

In fact, I hope that you've already had a few aha moments as you've read the preceding chapters. I've had a few revelations myself in the course of writing this book. Learning, as the sages say, is an ongoing process. But in all my years of teaching people about healthy cooking and living, the one outstanding lesson I've learned is that when people understand food and how it is affecting them, they can and do change their eating patterns more easily.

When you understand the *why*, you are equipped to make the choices of *how* you want to live and *what* you want to achieve for yourself, your family and the world.

The following chapter is intended to be a crash course in lifesaving that starts with understanding the fundamentals of nutrition; on how and what you eat has an impact on who you are and what will become of you.

I am focusing first on basic nutrition—but I'll make it as fun to read as possible. Since most readers new to vegan eating do have lots of questions about getting proper nutrition when they choose to eliminate animal products from their diets, it's the best place to start. Then I move into the "danger zone" foods or what Harry Potter fans might call the "dementors" of the food world because they'll suck the life out of you—meat, dairy, eggs and sugar. (I thought I'd save all the real yummy stuff about specific health-giving foods—their value, how to prepare and eat them—for chapter 5, "Eat Well for Life.")

SAY HELLO TO NUTRIENTS

To make the best food choices, you need to appreciate the underlying quality of food and what it does for you on the most basic level. There isn't a diet or health book around that doesn't talk about the big issues: protein, carbs, fat, fiber, etc. But, as you expect, we are going to be rethinking everything you thought you knew about these really important subjects. Depending on your level of interest and education, you might have heard some of this before. But don't assume anything. You know what that does…

Let's start with the most contentious issue when it comes to vegetarian and vegan lifestyle and my personal favorite—protein.

Protein: The Mighty Mouse Nutrient

"How can vegans get enough protein to be really healthy?"

I'm a mind reader. Actually, it's just a parlor trick I picked up from years of teaching and being asked this same question and its many variations: "How can I get protein into my diet if I cut out meat, dairy and eggs?"

Although protein is essential to our health, we have become completely unhinged on the topic. We are obsessed by the notion that we're not getting enough and always need more, more, more. The truth is that the human body requires only about 15 to 25% of its nutrients to be protein—and that's for very active types. So relax, will ya?

Let's make it easy to understand and apply to your new way of life, so you have no more questions about this one. First, remember that there is protein in everything you eat (except fruit), so the chances of not getting what you need (unless you are a fruititarian) are slim. Plus, it's important to remember that next to water, protein is the most plentiful substance in the body, with 60 to 70% of it housed in our skeletal muscles.

Let's say you are eating a diet of 1,600 to 1,800 calories a day so that you can lose some weight (remembering that about 2,000 calories a day will maintain your current weight, so to lose you need to slash some calories). Let's also say that you're exercising regularly, so you want to make sure that you are getting enough of this valuable nutrient, so that your protein is not stored for energy. That only increases your protein needs. On average, you need 20% of your calories to come from protein. That's 360 calories of your intake or 90 grams (since there are 4 calories in a gram of protein). So with a simple bit of math, you can see where your calories are coming from and how to utilize them to your advantage.

Let's take a look at some vegan sources of protein and their respective calorie counts for ½ cup or 4 ounces:

lentils	80
chickpeas	135
cannellini beans	150
black beans	114
tofu	79

Compare the above with a single ounce of extra-lean raw ground beef at 60 calories. One measly 6-ounce burger at 360 calories (from 90 grams) and you are all in for your protein calories for the day. And you know that people eat way more than that in one day. It's just another way that eating a crazy vegan diet gives you a leg up. Including beans or bean products at two of your meals, protein in snacks, as well as the protein that naturally exists in whole grains and veggies and you can see that it is a total no-brainer to get the protein you need, eat well and keep your calories in line with your goals. Of course, as you grow more and more active, your protein needs may increase, but you can easily adjust and eat accordingly.

A little protein goes a long way to do its job to build new tissue and repair what is torn apart. It's not a very efficient energy source but it's perfect to slow hunger and build strength.

Nothing keeps us feeling satisfied longer than protein. Protein-rich foods keep us from binge eating, because it makes us feel satisfied. Discovering this fact was huge for me and key to my own success. Before I figured out the protein thing, I craved, craved, craved sweets all the time. And

The Myth of Incomplete Protein

As much as I love Frances Moore Lappé's book *Diet for a Small Planet*, I hate the myth that it started, which plagues vegetarians and vegans to this day. The myth: That we can not, without seriously detailed protein combining, be properly nourished.

Most experts, including Drs. Neal Barnard, John McDougall and T. Colin Campbell, now debunk the idea of protein combining and state that simply eating a varied vegetarian or vegan diet with a balance of protein, fat and carbohydrate, with sufficient caloric intake provides more than enough protein.

Complete animal protein is not superior, as was previously believed, to protein made complete by coming from more than one source. It gives the same result in different ways and in fact is advantageous since it does not bring the baggage of saturated fat, excess calories, toxic residues and an overabundance of protein, which stresses the kidneys.

The average American consumes two to six times more protein than they require—and usually from animal products, with unfortunate results. So maybe we can finally stop worrying about this one.

did I mention that I craved sweets? The absolute second that I introduced proper levels of protein in my diet, the cravings ended. And while I have to admit that I still love sweets, I don't crave them anymore.

SOURCES OF PROTEIN

There are so many sources of protein in this crazy vegan life that you'll wonder if it's really so crazy after all. You already know about the weird "health" foods that contain lots of protein like tofu, tempeh (and all manner of soy products), beans, seeds and nuts. But now you can count whole grains and vegetables as a viable source of protein. These will also add variety to your diet, which is essential for a whole bunch of other reasons we'll talk about in the coming chapters.

Cows eat grass and they're not deficient in protein and last I looked, they don't do a lot of food combining!

I know what you're thinking: "I am not a cow!" Good point. But it makes sense that if any living creature can obtain its proper nutrients from plant

sources, then why not humans? Are we less evolved than our fellow creatures when it comes to digestion? (You can go back and read that bit about
our ancient ancestors in chapter 1.) And yes, I know that cows are built
digestively different from us. But the easiest and most convincing way to
demonstrate how much protein is available to us from plants compared to
meat is with the accompanying chart, which gives you a quick overview of
the protein content of a variety of foods, including meat, chicken, fish, nuts,
seeds, beans, vegetables and grains.

At first glance, this chart may seem misleading. One has to eat about
three times the amount of beans to get the same about of protein as, say,
from meat or chicken. But take a look at the numbers for nuts and seeds
compared with meat. They are pretty close. And yes, there are more calories from some of the non-meat choices, but the reality is that no one eats
only one ounce of chicken, meat or fish. But you would only eat an ounce of
nuts, if that much, so you need to put things into proper perspective. (Most
professional nutritionists consider about 4 ounces to be an average portion
size—and most people eat way more than that.) So while calorie for calorie
you may be getting more protein with animal food, it comes at the cost
of the fat, cholesterol and some other unsavory characters like pesticides,
antibiotics and whatnot that come along for the ride with animal protein.
At the end of the day, a vegetarian diet is far less calorically dense than any
meat-based diet. Period.

In addition to the plant-based sources of protein, samples of which
appear in the following chart, there are lots of meat substitutions available.
Some of these are great and provide plenty of plant protein but you have
to read the nutrition labels carefully to make sure that there's nothing in
these packaged veggie burgers, lunch "meats" or breakfast links that you
might not want to ingest. If you can't identify—or pronounce—an ingredient, perhaps there is a food choice that you can make that is more…well,
natural.

Just keep in mind that on any given day if you eat a salad with ¼ cup
of sunflower seeds (10 grams protein), a 4-ounce baked tofu sandwich on
whole grain bread (12.4 grams protein), a 10-ounce bowl of millet-vegetable
soup (10 grams protein), then you've racked up 34 grams of protein (about
32% of your daily needs) in one simple meal.

You and Your Protein

FOOD ITEM	QUANTITY	PROTEIN (GS)	CALORIES
Almonds	1 ounce (20–24 nuts)	6	160
Black turtle beans	1 ounce	2	11
Cannellini	1 ounce	4.25	13
Chicken breast	1 ounce	7.5	35
Chickpeas	1 ounce	1.7	11
Egg	1 large	50	75
Flaxseeds	1 ounce	5	95
Ground beef (17% fat)	1 ounce	7.11	66
Hazelnuts	1 ounce (18–20 nuts)	4	180
Lentils	1 ounce	4.5	11
Low-fat cottage cheese	1 ounce	3.1	35
Low-fat milk (1%)	1 ounce	3.5	11
Millet	1 ounce	2.5	34
Peanuts	1 ounce (28)	7	170
Pine nuts	1 ounce	7	160
Pumpkin seeds	1 ounce	5.3	154
Quinoa	1 ounce	1	34
Salmon	1 ounce	7.1	55
Soybeans	1 ounce	7.25	11
Soynuts	1 ounce	10	120
Sunflower seeds	1 ounce (20–25 nuts)	5	162
Tempeh	1 ounce	3	35
Tofu	1 ounce	3.1	35
Walnuts	1 ounce (14 halves)	4	190

Too Much of a Good Thing

When the body consumes more protein than it needs, poisons are created. Animal foods, the most popular source of protein in our modern culture, are highly unstable. Animal foods decompose rapidly and become toxic, which results in a virtual plethora of poisons being created in the body. From uric acid to sulfates to toxic bacteria, animal protein creates an internal environment akin to a trash-filled landfill. Remember that protein is rich in nitrogen, which, when broken down in the liver, creates ammonia...which is poisonous. When you eat more protein than you need, increased ammonia can harm cells and slow your day-to-day organ functions, which slows you way down...and not in a relaxed, Virgin Island vacation kind of way. More like a lethargic, dull kind of slow. Not only that, but excess protein robs the body of vitamin B_6 and calcium, causing the kidneys to be overworked. And we all know what happens when our kidneys overwork. We are exhausted, foggy and not very likely to be sharp in our decision making. All we want to do is sit and find some comfort.

However, eating the proper amount of protein for you makes you feel strong and vital, with focus like a heat-seeking missile. Your organs are functioning at their peak. Your tissue is being renewed and repaired at a normal, healthy rate. You are strong, happy, capable and confident.

And while vegetables are not what we think of when we think of growing muscle, it's time to rethink that notion. While no match for beans and bean products, fresh vegetables all provide some protein to add to our mix of daily fare. With corn, green peas and artichokes leading the pack with 4 grams of protein for each ½ cup serving, vegetables help to round out your protein needs so you can stay big and strong. None of the most commonly consumed veggies comes in at under 1 gram of protein for every ½ cup serving, so best to think twice before teasing that vegan colleague of yours. He or she could kick your butt...in the gym, of course. Most of us are pacifists and would never do such a thing.

Carbohydrates: Energy to Burn

There's so much nonsense out there about carbohydrates that I could fill a book with the myths and misinformation. Here are two of my favorites:

Myth: *High-carb diets increase your risk of heart disease, raising choles-terol and triglycerides and reducing HDL cholesterol.*

Truth: Well, sure this might be true if the carbs are refined (or *simple*) like white sugar, and if you consistently overeat. When people eat diets that include *complex carbohydrates*, like those found in whole grains, cholesterol levels fall, triglycerides normalize and they lose weight.

Myth: *Athletes, average gym rats and weekend warriors perform bet-ter and grow bigger muscle when they eat a high-protein, high-fat diet. Diets rich in carbohydrates inhibit the performance of any type of athlete, pro or amateur.*

Truth: The reality is that carbohydrate, not fat, is the primary fuel for strenuous exercise. Remember that fat only becomes available for fuel after twenty minutes of continuous exercise, so you must rely on carbs to fuel you for that first period of your hourlong workout (you are working out for an hour, right?). After your glycogen stores are depleted, then you burn body fat. Almost every study of athletes (professional and amateur) shows that consuming carbohydrates before and during an event improves performance. Consuming carbohydrates after an event replenishes glycogen (sugar) stores for your next challenge.

OH, CARBS, POOR CARBS

They've been vilified and shunned. Some people—fitness gurus and reg-ular folks alike—even think that carbs should be labeled with the skull and crossbones, especially when it comes to weight loss. Think again! Carbohy-drate energy is your key to finding your ideal weight and staying there. But it's not just about the carbs; it's about the *kind* of carbs. (More on this later...)

Carbohydrates are the primary source of fuel for many of your organs, including your brain, central nervous system and kidneys. Your digestive tract breaks the carbs into glucose, while the pancreas secretes insulin to help the sugar move from your blood to your cells, producing fuel. And when you are eating right that happens with amazing efficiency.

The unfounded belief that carbohydrates cause weight gain is deeply misleading. The truth is that you gain weight from too many calories taken in and not enough expended. A diet rich in whole grains, beans and their byproducts, vegetables and fruit with moderate amounts of good fat and no animal protein is your best shot at losing weight and maintaining a healthy body.

Let me try to set you straight on the whole low-carb thing. Carb-restricted diets work; they really do. But they work because they restrict your total caloric intake. Every one of those plans deprives your body of the nutrients it needs and causes major metabolic disturbances. Ouch! There really is nothing special about the proportion of protein to carbohydrate. When your calories are highly restricted, you'll lose weight. The problem is that most people can't stay with these plans long-term. (Read more about high-protein/low-carb diets in chapter 5.)

If your body doesn't get enough carbohydrate fuel for energy, it turns to stored fat and muscle protein. Your body must have energy. It will take it from wherever it's available. But at some point in this process, your body moves into a state of ketosis, a common condition among people who are starving, anorexia nervosa patients, people suffering from untreated insulin-dependent diabetes—and people on high–animal protein diets. There is also growing evidence that the heart can't function at its optimum when ketones are its main source of energy. Plus, ketosis can cause kidney and liver damage by turning your blood highly acidic, and it gives you dry skin *and* bad breath! Do you care now?

ALL CARBS ARE NOT CREATED EQUAL

We need carbs for energy; ultimately, glucose is the fuel that we operate on. But all carbohydrates are not the same. When you eat *simple carbohy-drates*, like white or refined sugar (in all its guises such as fructose and those other names ending in "ose," which rhymes with gross), white bread, white pasta, potatoes or white rice, your glucose levels shoot up like a rocket and you feel great—for about twenty minutes. These kinds of carbs bypass the small intestines, dump right into the bloodstream, and instantly alter your blood chemistry. Then your pancreas gets the message to release insulin (the hormone that regulates sugar levels in the blood) to stabilize your blood sugar. If this becomes your habit (there's that word again), then too much insulin is secreted on a regular basis and your glucose levels drop quickly and significantly. You crash and burn, and are left feeling jittery, tired and cranky. And guess what? You seek out more sugar for energy and the vicious cycle continues. Kicking sugary foods out of your life can very well be the key to ridding yourself of everyday crankiness, not to mention the onset of type 2 diabetes. Studies have shown that people who dump the sugar habit have even gotten substantial relief from symptoms of depression, with the bonus benefit of having more sustained energy, vitality, clearer thinking, a stronger immune function and normal body weight. You don't have to be Einstein to make this equation work: simple carbohydrates = empty calories = poor health and a fat body. Got it?

Whole grains, or complex carbs, on the other hand, nourish and fuel your body while keeping blood sugar level. And emotionally? Well, no more roller coasters; you can save those for the amusement park. Whole grains are high in fiber and are composed of long-chain molecules. Too much science? Just remember this: whole grains like brown rice, quinoa, millet,

Measuring the Effect of Carbs

You may have heard of the Glycemic Index (GI). This system, designed for use by doctors and nutritionists, can help you decide how to choose proper carbs for your diet. The GI measures the relative rate at which a food will raise blood glucose. Foods are measured against pure glucose—or nice, white, refined sugar—which has been given the score of 100. (It's sort of like golf—the lower the score, the better.) Quick-hit, high-GI foods are those with scores of 70 or more. Foods that take longer to be absorbed into the bloodstream are given a score of 55 or lower, are considered to be low-GI foods and are generally healthier choices.

You can probably guess that low-GI foods include nuts, whole grains, whole grain bread, beans, soy products, most vegetables and some fruit. Medium-GI foods include sugar (with a GI of 65, so it's on the high side of medium) and orange juice (with a GI of 55), while high-GI foods include potatoes, white bread and white rice (with GIs of 89, 72, and 79, respectively).

Now, before you make yourself crazy searching out the GI of every food you eat, remember that the GI is easily influenced by food combinations. For instance, adding protein to a meal decreases the impact that a food has to raise blood glucose levels. Or adding sugar to a whole grain cereal will raise the GI of the dish. There are lots of sources of GI information on the Internet and in books, but there's no need to search through the charts and tables and make detailed calculations to make smart choices. As a rule of thumb, choose whole, unrefined grains, beans, vegetables, some fruit and skip the "white" foods: refined flour, sugar, white potatoes—oh, and milk!

barley, oats, whole wheat pasta and breads break down and release slowly into the bloodstream, providing a steady stream of energy for us to count on, like having your burners on "simmer" all the time. No more ups and downs in our moods or our energy because we always have resources to draw on.

How much whole grain makes for a healthy choice, particularly if you are looking to drop a clothing size or two? Ideally, you want five servings a day of these valuable and yummy foods. That's not as much as it sounds. One serving equals 1 cup of cooked whole wheat pasta; ½ cup of uncooked oatmeal, brown rice, millet, barley or quinoa; a 4-ounce sweet potato; one ear of fresh corn; or a slice of whole grain bread.

A BITTER ADDICTION

While sugar is *orgasmically* delicious, it will make you fat and it will kill you—slowly, painfully. Simple sugars create anything but a happy ending for our health. Those sparkling little white or brown crystals, high-fructose corn syrup (the Darth Vader of food), maple syrup, organic cane juice, date sugar, turbinado sugar, raw sugar and refined fruit juices are simple carbohydrates, composed of loosely bound molecules of glucose. These are unlike complex carbohydrates, which are composed of tightly bound chains of glucose molecules. The difference in our bodies is like night and day. And as usual, the problem lies not in the sugar itself, but in the amount of simple carbohydrates that we consume versus the amount of complex carbohydrates.

Sugar is found, of course, in the obvious places: candies, chocolate bars, soft drinks and other snack foods. And if you are thinking that you don't eat any of that, well, just read a few labels. Sugar is an ingredient in so many other products, from breads and pasta to cereals to salad dressings and sauces and other processed foods, often disguised with names that you don't recognize as sugar. In this case you do have to be a rocket scientist to decipher all the code names. But as the saying goes, "A rose by any other name..." When you eat processed foods, you are consuming tremendous amounts of simple, refined sugar. If you add fast food to the equation, you eat a whopping forty-nine pounds of sugar each year. That's a lot of sweet going around!

And if you think shopping in a natural foods store is safe, think again. In most cases, you'll need to read labels as diligently as you do in any supermarket. From maple syrup, fructose, sucrose, molasses, maltose and organic cane juice (which is just a fancy name designed to disguise sugar), many natural products contain as much simple sugar as any processed snack. There are not any chemical additives or colorings or preservatives and that's good, but there could be a lot more simple sugar in those "healthy snacks" than you want to eat.

The molecular structure of simple sugars causes them to be rapidly absorbed into the bloodstream, which causes the glucose level to rise very quickly. As I just said, when this happens, the pancreas (the organ that regulates blood sugar) secretes insulin that moves excess sugar from the blood to the cells. With this, blood sugar drops, resulting in rapid fluctuations in metabolism—what we know as sugar "highs" and "lows," as the levels of glucose in the blood rise and fall erratically. We experience a burst of energy as the levels of glucose rise followed by the inevitable crash as the glucose levels drop, leaving us feeling depleted and tired. Eventually, we become hypoglycemic and over time, type 2 diabetes becomes a real threat, especially if we are also eating saturated fats from animal foods.

If we continue this pattern over time, the body grows exhausted from the extreme levels of energy, as well as the sugar robbing our bones, teeth and skin of essential minerals, with the loosening of tissue and muscle, leaving us looking weak and puffy—not to mention overweight and lethargic. There is no way to sugarcoat this information, I'm afraid.

By the way, if you are looking for ways to cut the sugar but keep some sweet in your diet, check out "A Very Sweet, Corny Story" (in the box that follows) and the section on artificial and alternative sweeteners later in this chapter for both the good and bad news.

MORE IS LESS

Let's end this section on carbs on a happy note with some good news: There are 6 calories in 1 gram of carbs (whether simple or complex) and 9 in a gram of fat. That may not seem like much of a difference, but think of it in terms of volume, not weight. A gram of carbs will have more volume than a gram of fat because of density. Look at it this way. One-half cup of cooked brown rice has 100 calories, 22 grams of carbs and 0.9 grams of fat. A single tablespoon of butter has 100 calories, 0 carbs and 12 grams of fat. Not much bang for your buck in the butter, you must admit. Add in the brown rice's high fiber benefit, which helps you feel full longer (not to

A Very Sweet, Corny Story

So maybe you thought I would be sharing one of those Moon-in-June, lovey-dovey romantic tales of young lovers in Iowa or Kansas. No, this is a story of our love affair with a sweetie named high-fructose corn syrup. It's a contemporary love story, full of highs and lows, and it ends rather badly.

High-fructose corn syrup, in use in food products since the early 1980s, now represents more than 40% of the sweeteners added to food and beverages on the market today. Interestingly, the epidemic rise in obesity can be traced back to the early '80s as well. And before you even think about citing the studies that asserts high-fructose corn syrup is the same calorically as sugar, think again. Although similar to sugar in calories, high-fructose corn syrup actually triggers overeating because it inhibits the secretion of the hormone leptin, the single element that signals that you are full and you should stop eating. Eating foods with high-fructose corn syrup can cause you to consume three hundred more calories than you need before your body gets the message that it has been fed at all!

In 1970, Americans were consuming about a pound of high-fructose corn syrup per year. As of 2004, we were consuming sixty-three pounds annually. That's 313 calories each and every day.

Every food producer knows the facts about high-fructose corn syrup— *every one*! So with the obesity problem growing at alarming rates, why is this insidious product still being used? Why not just use simple sugar? Even with all of its problems, sugar is more natural for us and would do less harm. But high-fructose corn syrup is cheaper—and it's subsidized by the federal government via the tariffs on sugar and direct subsidies to corn growers.

While the original intention of farm subsidies was to help farmers thrive in tough times, along the way even the best intentions, as they say, paved the road to perdition.

Most of the high-fructose corn syrup is made by Archer Daniels Midland, a behemoth of a corporation that has been the largest recipient of the corn subsidy dollars—more than $41.9 billion between 1994 and 2004. And in case you are wondering, you and I pay for those subsidies with our tax dollars. So let's get this straight: A huge, multibillion-dollar corporation has figured out a way to steal dollars intended for average farmers, and we pay for it with taxes. And the corporation makes huge profits from a product that is killing us . . . bite by bite!

mention keeping your intestines healthy), and you have a winning ingredient in carbohydrates.

Rethink carbs before it's too late.

Fat Chance

Fat has gotten a very bad reputation. It's become like the "gangsta" of all food groups. The truth about fat may surprise you—and delight you more than a little bit.

Dietary fats play important roles in maintaining a healthy body of normal weight. Fats make our skin and hair gloriously healthy; they provide insulation and regulate body temperature; they help balance hormones and cell membrane development. So you must, must, must eat them.

But before you throw a fat party, keep on reading. Excess consumption of fat, particularly the saturated and trans fat types can throw your health into a tailspin and make the numbers on the scale skyrocket.

The standard American diet is hardly healthy when it comes to fat consumption, with more than 50% of daily calories coming from fat. That's twice what it should be. And while no healthy diet suggests cutting fats completely out of the picture, you need to limit them to 30% or less of your daily fare if you are to preserve your health—particularly that of your heart—and if you are to find your way to a normal weight and stay there.

Read labels carefully and understand what fats will serve you best and how to use them as keys to managing this essential nutrient.

FATS TO SKIP

The single worst fat—the skull and crossbones—is *trans fats*. These fats used to occur naturally only in meats. But then the food industry, in their ceaseless quest to fatten their bottom lines, even at the expense of our bottoms and waists, decided to chemically alter vegetable oils to lengthen their shelf life and give food a more appetizing mouth feel. These fats, which are directly linked to heart disease, some cancer, type 2 diabetes and obesity, are found in everything from packaged cookies to salad dressings. They will kill you... and the process won't be pretty.

But wait! Haven't trans fats been banned? Even KFC advertises that there are no trans fats in their buckets of goodies. So we're safe from harm, right? Not so fast. According to a 2006 report out of Brandeis University, the ingredient now used to replace trans fats may be just as bad, or worse, for your health. Known as *interesterified fats* or *stearate-rich fats* (a chemically processed saturated fatty acid that is replacing some of the polyunsaturated fats in oils to make it neutral and solidify oil or fat), this new substitute has been shown to decrease HDL (good) cholesterol and increase blood sugar by 20%, substantially boosting the risk of heart disease. This alternative to trans fats can do just as much damage, maybe more.

Next on the hit parade are *saturated fats*. Found in all animal products, saturated fats are difficult for the body to break down, which makes them hang around in your blood and stick to the walls of your veins and arteries. Like their cousins, trans fats, they are directly linked to heart disease and cancer. And you also want to skip the veggie versions of saturated fats, too, like coconut oil and palm oil. I know they are the new darlings of the natural products industry, especially coconut oil. But in my opinion, they are still saturated fats and I think that we have all eaten way too many of those anyhow. For me, the jury is still out on these two oils, so use them at your own risk.

FATS TO ENJOY

If the idea of "good" fat comes as a surprise to you, you must have been living under a rock for a while. Welcome back to the world. The best fats for you to enjoy are monounsaturated and polyunsaturated fats and essential fatty acids (EFAs). They are dramatically very different from trans, saturated and interesterified fats, and they benefit your health in different ways.

Monounsaturated fats come to us in olives and extra virgin olive oil. (You get all the benefits of the antioxidants as well as healthy fat from this first press oil.) They also come from avocado oil, macadamia nut oil, walnut, almond, hazelnut and peanut oils. Soybean oil is also a monounsaturated fat, but the quality and flavor are often second-rate to the other options. *Polyunsaturated fats* include canola, corn, sunflower, safflower and sesame seed oils. Omega-3s, while also abundant in fish, are found in flaxseed, hempseed and chia seed oil for us vegans. (More on omega-3s on page 62.)

Monounsaturated oils are the best for cooking as they remain stable under heat, but are easily digested and converted into energy by your body. Poly's, as I call them, are wonderfully healthy oils, but can only be cooked for short times at lower heats to maintain their health benefits. I tend to use them more for baking and less for high heat. (The one exception here is corn oil. There are no organic versions that I have found and with the extensive genetic modifying of our commercial corn crops being what it is, I am not taking the chance of supporting that with my money. And there are so many yummy options, I don't need to…and you don't either.)

One of the main cautions that I'll offer about fats is that you have to be careful with foods that you don't prepare yourself—packaged foods and restaurant fare. So many dishes, even the ones labeled as "healthy" have fats hidden in places you can't imagine…to say nothing of excess sodium and sugar, so look before you eat. Check labels; in a restaurant, ask how foods are cooked, as very often even the vegetable side dishes are cooked in butter or the vegetable soups have meat or chicken stock as the base. A simple Caesar salad can have more fat than a cheeseburger. So much for healthy!

Is Fat Making Us Fat?

As you've probably figured out, I love to dispel a myth or two. And here's one of my favorites: Eating fat doesn't make you fat. The thinking is that we're consuming less fat today than we did ten years ago yet we're still getting fatter, so dietary fat must not be to blame. It must be something else. The truth is that we're consuming a little more fat now than before. But fat is not the only culprit in the battle of the bulge. Already in the best chemical form for storage, fat is almost effortlessly transferred to our body's fat cells. This transfer is so easy and smooth that the chemical structure of the dietary fat remains largely unchanged as it is stored. So when you eat too much of it, it stores beautifully on your hips, thighs, butt, back, upper arms and tummy.

On average, people daily consume 250 more calories of refined flours and sugars than they did fifteen years ago. Because of the added refined carbohydrates, the *percentage* of fat in the diet may have been reduced between 1980 and 1990, but the actual grams or amount of fat consumed has remained the same or risen. On top of that, Americans eat more calories than needed: on average, 3,500 calories per day. The average woman needs 1,800 to 2,000, while men need 2,000 to 2,400 to function as well-fed humans. The reason for the rise in obesity is no mystery—Americans eat a high-calorie, high-fat diet and do not get enough exercise.

So sure, fat is a problem, but overeating and undermoving is bigger.

ESSENTIAL FATTY ACIDS

EFAs, as they are affectionately known in the food world, are unsaturated fats that are essential to human health, but cannot be manufactured in the body. There are two major types of EFAs: omega-3 and omega-6. These fats are responsible for so many of our body's functions, from metabolism to heart health to nervous system function, hence the word *essential*.

So while you certainly need to be aware of the amount of fat you eat, you need, need, need to eat some fat if you are to find your way to your ideal weight and glowing, vital health. It's the *kind* of fat that's important.

Essential fatty acids not only reduce the risk of heart disease, but they also can lift your spirits. Studies show that people eating omega-3-rich foods show a 50% reduction in symptoms of depression and they often show the improvement within hours of eating them!

Not only beneficial to your mood, EFAs are vital to the long-term maintenance of human tissue, promoting the healthy function of our brain, heart, digestive and immune systems. The ideal balance of these essential fats is one key to our health. The recommended ratio, three parts omega-6 to one part omega-3, is not as easy to obtain as it sounds.

Omega-6 is very common, found in most foods from meat and dairy products to veggies, bean, nuts and seeds. We really have no problem getting enough omega-6, unless we are eating a very low-fat diet. Omega-6 is needed for blood clotting, proper circulation, healthy kidney and liver function and proper healing of internal injury. However, since it's abundantly found in most people's diets, there isn't much worry about getting it. Once again, it's about balance.

Omega-3 is a less commonly available fatty acid. Found only in fish and some vegetables, nuts and seeds, the effects of omega-3 deficiencies are becoming an epidemic in our modern world. Although we need only small amounts of this powerful essential fat, it is responsible for all vital body functions, including the fluidity of our blood, increased immune function, balance of cholesterol production, proper growth, fetal development, mental acuity and cell renewal. A deficiency of omega-3 can cause such problems as arrhythmia, asthma, arteriosclerosis, attention deficit disorder, bipolar disorder, breast cancer, colon cancer, diabetes, hypertension, inflammation, immune disorder, migraine headaches, obesity, prostate cancer and psoriasis...to name but a few!

Essential fatty acids make blood platelets less sticky, so they don't cause hardening of the arteries, like trans fat and saturated fat. Essential fatty acids are too important to the body to be used for mere energy storage, like the other fats, so they are more quickly used and do not land on our hips so easily. They also help carry toxins from the skin, kidneys, lungs and intestinal tract, and create energy within the cells by delivering oxygen from red blood cells. Essential fatty acids are made into the hormone prostaglandin, which controls cholesterol production.

The latest information available to us about omega-3 is nothing short of amazing. Regular consumption of this essential fat helps the body to burn more fat calories in a day. One of the most important aspects of these findings is that omega-3, by burning more fat calories, results in reduced insulin production. Insulin reduces the use of fat for fuel while promoting fat storage in the presence of excess calories. Insulin increases the activity of a hormone that stores fat and inhibits the production of lipase, the enzyme that breaks stored fat to be used as energy. Oh, and it aids in the conversion of carbohydrate to fat. Now do you see why you don't want high levels of insulin running around in your blood?

For vegetarians and vegans, sources of omega-3 are scarce. With trace amounts in avocados, walnuts and pumpkin seeds, many have looked to flaxseeds and flaxseed oil, hempseeds and hempseed oil, as well as chia seeds and chia seed oil and other supplements. (My personal favorite is a line of flax oil blends called Heart Shape, which combines flax with olive and sunflower oils. You can cook with them without harming the omega-3s.) Fish, well-known to be high in EFAs, doesn't have to be the answer. And as our waterways grow more polluted and farming practices more compromised, I believe that fish will become a very controversial food for us.

Whether or not you grasp the science of fat, it's easy see that without the right fats in our diet, good health is more difficult to maintain. The body has difficulty absorbing fat-soluble nutrients so vital to good health, such as vitamin D and calcium. So don't be so quick to adopt the latest no-fat craze. Instead, eat the appropriate fat for your needs and discover for yourself the key to good health and vitality.

Fiber Is Your Friend

Fiber fills you up, period. Eating foods that are high in fiber make you feel like you are eating a ton, but without a ton of calories. Fiber-rich foods travel through the digestive system more slowly, so you get to keep that comfy full feeling longer. You're not always foraging for food, grazing your way to obesity. Fiber is a win-win for you all around. You get full faster; stay full longer; keep your intestines functioning at their peak so you are assimilating nutrients with great efficiency and helping to prevent colon cancer.

Ah, but I can hear your big excuse already: "High-fiber veggies make me *musical*." Well, here's the deal. Changing up from a standard American junk food diet to one that is rich in vegetables, fruits and whole grains immediately ups your fiber intake—a lot. For some of you, with digestion weakened from years of consuming saturated fat, sugar, additives and other chemicals in processed foods, that can be a bit of a shock to your system. See, there's a gas-producing bacteria needed by the intestines to break down fiber, which can result in you becoming your own "musical accompaniment." But your body is a miracle. Within two to three weeks, your intestines adjust to this new amount of fiber and things settle down, so to speak.

One more thing: When I was studying Chinese medicine, my teacher once said of digestion that there are no teeth in the intestines, only in the mouth. It was his way of saying that the process of digestion begins in the mouth with chewing, as saliva is produced to begin to break down food before it hits the digestive tract. The key to great digestion is not in the pharmacy, but in the chewing.

So grab some veggie sticks, a piece of fruit (but not a whole bowl), and whole grain cereals like oatmeal, brown rice, quinoa and popcorn, and you will sail through the day. Skip right over the cookies, cakes and the rest of those snacks made from white flour and sugar. They'll make you ravenously hungry and steal your health, but not before they make you fat.

The Skinny on Salt

While a necessary ingredient to life, salt has two very different sides to its nature. Vital to our existence, natural sea salt is rich in trace minerals and sodium chloride, which are necessary to the health of our blood. On the other hand, there's processed, refined table salt...the kind found on the table at the local diner, in junk foods like potato chips, popcorn and salted nuts, and in processed foods and meats. Commercial table salt, far removed from its natural state in the sea, has been stripped of nutrients, reenriched and laced through with chemicals and preservatives. Even small amounts of table salt will have a most dramatic effect on our blood chemistry and organ health. Table salt will kill you.

Why use salt at all? Do we need it? What is its job? Applied to food in cooking, salt causes contraction, sealing in the flavor of each ingredient while forcing liquid from the food, intensifying the taste. That's why you miss it so much when it's not there. Salt works similarly in the body. Consumption of natural salt in appropriate quantities aids the body in staying strong, with healthy blood, as your muscles and body tissue contract slightly. Used well, natural salt can also help your skin hold moisture and retain its elasticity and firmness.

However, inappropriate use of salt or poor-quality salt will cause tissue in the body to tighten and constrict, inhibiting the flow of blood to our various organs. Energy flow is blocked and you begin to feel tightening throughout the body. Your muscles begin to contract, growing stiff and hard. Your blood pressure rises and your veins and arteries stiffen. Your body, desperately dehydrated, holds on to moisture in the form of water retention. You grow stiff, sore and puffy with edema.

Over time, should excessive use of salt continue, you will also see signs of degeneration in your bones. Salt can dry the body, inhibiting the absorption of vitamins essential to bone health and strength. You will lose your ability to stand tall and straight as your bones grow brittle and weak.

So are you doomed to a life of eating meals that are flat, with no taste and no sparkle? Of course not. Light to moderate use of salt in cooking not only adds to the pleasure of eating food, but starts the process of digestion, causing the food to soften as you apply cooking heat. Natural, unrefined sea salt, naturally aged soy sauce and miso are the best choices for use of salt. That being said, the old rule holds true: no sprinkling salt or soy sauce on cooked food at the table. It never really becomes a part of the flavor of the dish and all you taste is salt. Raw salt will make your muscles tight and hard, your skin dry, your joints inflexible and your fingers, toes, face and ankles puffy with water retention. Used delicately in cooking, salt makes eating a pleasure, your blood healthy, your muscles strong and your skin firm and elastic.

Iron, Man

When we think of iron, we think of "pumping it" much more than eating it. This mineral, which is essential to your health, works as the key oxygen carrier in your blood. Should your iron levels not be up to par, shall we say, you will experience fatigue, lethargy, insomnia and an inability to concentrate that leaves you feeling "bone tired." And we all know how likely you are to stay on a health and fitness plan when you feel beat.

But you don't need to have a steak to get the iron you need...or a burger, chicken or cheese, although the iron in these foods is easily absorbed by your body. The truth is the truth, even when I don't like it. You can, however, get what you need to feel well, vital and strong (1.8 milligrams daily) from whole grains, vegetables, fruit and nuts. Remember, though, you must get vitamin C along with the iron to get the bang for your buck that you want. Wheat, millet, oats, brown rice, broccoli, kale, spinach, collard greens, asparagus, dried beans, prunes, dried apricots and raisins are some of the richest sources of iron in the plant kingdom and since they are also sources of vitamin C, you win on all fronts. There are also iron supplements on the market to help boost your iron levels, should you need them. Only a blood test will reveal your iron needs, so don't play doctor. Work with one and get a real view of your blood and what is going on.

One little nutrient and you feel great, are incredibly strong and awake, haven't contributed to your own heart disease and obesity by eating meat and you have become an iron man or woman. Makes sense to me.

Folate: It's Easy Being Leafy Green

There is not a vegetable on earth that you should not enjoy and love with all your heart (you heart will thank you...), but of all the vegetables that Mother Nature has so lovingly provided, green leafies take the prize as the most precious to your body.

It's late in the afternoon and you need a snack to keep your energy up. But wait—before you pop open that bag of potato chips or tear into that candy bar, consider a bowl of kale instead. Hang on a sec, and give me a minute to get you past your immediate reaction, which is probably "Yuck!" What are you hoping that snack will do? Give you a little pick-me-up? Cut the hunger pangs? Focus your mind on the task at hand...or give you a diversion from a boring bit of work?

Personally, I always used to reach for something sweet to lift my energy in the afternoon before I "hurt somebody," as I used to say. I used to experience such a drop in my energy that everything and everyone irritated me. You know that feeling. Switching up to greens instead of candy changed everything for me. It will for you, too.

Dark leafy greens, like kale, collard greens, spinach, broccoli and even Romaine lettuce are rich sources of folate, a B vitamin that supports the production of serotonin, a brain chemical that helps to stabilize your mood.

One study has shown that close to 38% of people who were feeling blue, with low energy and lack of focus had low levels of folate, while another study revealed that depressed people experienced improved moods when they ate folate-rich foods like greens.

Even bitter greens, like broccoli rabe, escarole, watercress and dandelion are not only delicious and help to stabilize moods but also have the added benefit of aiding the liver in its job of metabolizing carbohydrates, fat and protein more efficiently, and helping to stabilize our weight.

You can never get enough greens in your diet, but in reality, it doesn't take much to get the mood-boosting benefits of folate. A mere 400 micrograms will do the trick for keeping you happy and energized, which translates to about 1 cup of loosely packed raw greens. Kale is the queen here, followed closely by spinach, collards, broccoli, Brussels sprouts and asparagus.

You may be saying that you don't need greens because you aren't depressed or blue at all. You feel just fine; thanks very much. Then consider this: Greens are an essential part of maintaining heart health and stabilizing your weight. Loaded with antioxidants, soluble fiber, and vitamins C, D and K, dark leafies are your best tools for maintaining vascular strength. And with kale having only 34 calories a cup, these delicate beauties will never land on your hips...even sautéed.

You may say that you can't just get up and steam a bowl of kale in your cubicle at 3 p.m., when you still have hours at the office. True. You can, however, take a couple of minutes in the morning or the night before and steam a few leaves; chop a few carrot pieces and stir it all together with a touch of olive oil and lemon juice. As it sits in the container, it marinates to create a lovely wilted salad. No more excuses.

And you thought that kale was just the garnish around a salad bar.

Black Beans, Bananas, and B$_6$

Just like our pal folate, vitamin B$_6$, also known as pyridoxine, helps your brain produce serotonin, the "feel-good" chemical. A deficiency in this essential compound has been linked to feeling "blue." According to research done at the University of Arizona Health Science Center, one in four people who are depressed are deficient in B vitamins. And all you need is 1.3 milligrams of this powerful little vitamin to feel better. A banana, ½ cup of oatmeal, ½ cup of cooked black beans or 1 cup of carrot sticks and you are there. If that is too much for you, simply take a supplement that provides at least 1.3 milligrams each day.

But it gets better with B_6. It works together with folic acid and vitamin B_{12} to stabilize homocysteine levels, reducing your risk of heart attack and stroke. And this water-soluble vitamin works in the body to convert protein to energy, making you feel big and strong.

Calcium and Your Bones, Your Weight... Your Everything

We all know from advertisements that calcium is essential to healthy bones. But did you know that getting enough calcium in your daily diet makes you happier? And did you know that it is one of the keys to help maintain a healthy weight? Oh, and it helps you concentrate and focus better. Calcium helps your muscles and nerves to perform better and your blood to clot better. Enzyme activities are increased. And it waxes your car. (Just kidding... wanted to see if you are paying attention. But, honestly it'll help you get that job done as well.)

When you feel down or low, instead of mindlessly picking up some comfort food snack like milk and cookies or ice cream, remember that calcium is the secret ingredient to helping you feel better. Clinical research at Columbia University has shown that maintaining proper levels of calcium in the body decreases moodiness substantially. And just 1,000 milligrams of calcium will do the trick.

But put down that glass of milk or that tub of ice cream. Despite what you have heard in ads, milk and dairy products are not your best sources of calcium. Sure, they have a ton of it, but what the ads forget to tell you (I am certain they forget; I mean, they wouldn't lie, right?) is that only 12 to 25% of the calcium in dairy products can be absorbed and used by your body. What you do get plenty of is saturated fat to make you fat and protein that leaches precious calcium from your bones! I guess the ad agency missed that part of the research!

Plant-based sources of calcium, like leafy greens, broccoli, Brussels sprouts and mustard greens have an absorption rate of 50 to 64%... double that of milk! And wait, there's more: These vegetables are rich sources of antioxidants, folates, phytochemicals, other essential vitamins and nutrients, fiber, iron and complex carbohydrates, with little or no saturated fat. So you get the calcium you need (an average 300 milligrams in 1 cup of cooked greens), in a form that your body can absorb and use, with no harm to your heart or your waistline.

How's your milk mustache looking now?

AND NOW FOR SOMETHING COMPLETELY DIFFERENT

You had to see it coming. With all the references to the ill effects of meat, dairy, chicken and eggs, you had to know that I would devote more than a few scary statistics to inspire the rethinking of your life.

The Big Four: meat, dairy, poultry and sugar substitutes are some of the greatest threats to the health of this country—and the world. I couldn't write this whole section on nutrition and not give you the facts of life, so to speak. It's one thing to espouse the wonders of kale; that's easy. It's quite another to take on the real truth about what meat, dairy, poultry and artificial sweeteners are doing to our collective health.

I truly believe that when people know better, they will do better. So here it is, the truth, as I know it, about the foods I consider to be unfit for human consumption.

The Meaty Truth

My father was a butcher so there was, of course, lots of meat on our family table. But from as far back as I can remember, I had trouble with it. I just didn't like it—not the smell, the texture, the taste. My dad said it was torture to watch me eat.

In high school at about the same time that I "came out" as a vegetarian, my father was offered the opportunity to make a bit of extra money by working for a few days in a slaughterhouse. He jumped at the chance for extra cash and so left early one Saturday morning for his "second" job. To our surprise he was home by noon. As we ran to greet him, we realized something was wrong. With a ghostly pallor and slumped shoulders, he was a far cry from the tall, strapping, healthy specimen of a man who'd left earlier that day. He walked past us with barely a word and went directly to my mother in the kitchen, where we found him sitting at the table, sobbing as though his heart would break.

"I couldn't do it," he said to my mother. I'll never forget those words. He then proceeded to tell her how he couldn't look into the eyes of the animals and then take their lives. I remember him telling her that you could see and even smell the fear of the doomed animals. For several months afterward, we were an experimental vegetarian family, with my mother joking that she would write a cookbook called 365 Things to Do with Broccoli. It didn't last, though. When the shock wore off my father, meat was back on the table. But I was changed forever. The thought of killing a living creature, especially one weaker than I, was unbearable to me. And while lots of things have changed in my life since then, my opinion that the human body doesn't need or thrive on meat hasn't.

Now hang on. This is not the part of the book where I go all "animal activist" on you. Sorry, fellow vegans, that's just not my thing. Studying macrobiotic cooking, I discovered a lot of things about food. One of the beautiful things about this philosophy is that the choices you make are based on understanding the energy of the food you are about to eat and determining if that choice serves you. It's not about morality and sentiment. It's about functioning at our optimum levels, so that we can fit easily and harmoniously into the environment, so that we can work together in peace and live happier lives, actually benefiting the environment by our presence, rather than being a part of the problem. Eating macrobiotically allows you to be a part of the life around you. Very often, that leads to vegan eating, since you do not wish to inflict harm or suffering on other beings.

Meat just doesn't fit the bill for humans. I *know* that meat has been a food choice throughout the world for ages. Animal foods have been used as part of man's diet in many cultures, in varying proportions. And I know that there has never been a traditional society that was totally vegetarian. And I know that you love meat. But the simple fact that we are so unhealthy and overweight has to speak for itself.

As humans, we simply aren't built to consume great quantities of meat. The structure of our intestines, stomach, teeth, even our skin is not designed to process and discharge meat without working our body incredibly hard. I'm not saying we don't ever digest meat; just that it makes us work hard in the process of assimilating it. We don't need meat in our diet as human beings...not for strength, not for energy, not for vitality. In fact, more often than not, we get just the opposite.

Meat is incredibly dense, composed of three basic ingredients: protein, water and fat, in varying amounts, depending on the animal. These proteins and fats are different from animal to animal and will behave differently in us. The conventional belief that protein is protein and fat is fat is simply not true. Each animal has its own unique makeup and this distinctive character is infused into every part of the animal, even the quality of its protein and fat.

Meat's structure is composed of long, thin cells that make up muscle tissue. Muscle tissues are bound together by thin but tough sheets of connective tissue, which group them together in bundles. The protein of meat is protein of movement, meaning that when they get the appropriate message from the animal's nervous system, the protein can propel it into action. When you eat meat, you are consuming tough fibers designed for movement, so your system has to work quite hard to digest it. As a result, eating meat robs your strength. When you eat calorically dense food, your intestines must draw energy from just about everywhere in the body in order to process it. That kind of effort, especially on a regular basis, keeps your body in high gear all the time and simply wears you out.

When you eat meat, you create a sort of internal friction with your intestines expanding and contracting during digestion. In fact, all of your organ functions move into overdrive. You produce a lot of heat, thereby producing a lot of energy. You can only use so much fuel. The body seeks release of excess energy, just as it seeks release in other ways. As heat builds internally, the body grows irritated and aggravated. Think about how you feel when the weather's hot and humid—cranky, irritable and lethargic. Put that feeling inside your body. Yikes! This energy can discharge in a variety of ways. Many people argue that it gives them strength. It's true that red meat was traditionally served to warriors. But to create what—a nice, even temperament to sit around the negotiating table? Meat creates excessive energy that shows itself in the form of aggression and quick tempers. Energy comes in quick, erratic bursts, instead of balanced, slow-releasing energy. And that was in the "old days," when the meat was the organic, free-range, Old MacDonald–farm meat that's being touted now as better for us. Today's commercially produced meat is another story…maybe another book. Nowadays you also get the "benefit" of antibiotics, growth hormones, pesticides and herbicides, from the environment and their feed. (But you read all about those in the first chapter…)

Meat makes your muscles bulky and tight, contracting the body, leaving little room for flexibility. Your body grows tired from overwork. Your nervous system is irritated because your liver is in overdrive trying to accommodate the excessive nutrition and energy. You seek more and more intense stimulation to open and relax your body, which often come in the form of hot spices and sugar. A layer of saturated fat builds up under your skin, literally desensitizing it to stimulation, causing you to require more and more intensity in your life. It's literally harder for us to feel things when we eat meat. It's exhausting just to think about that kind of energy.

Fowl Play

I know; I know: chicken's healthier. Right? Every diet plan since the dawn of diet plans says so. Sorry, kids.

Chickens have very different eating and digestive patterns than we do. With no teeth, food passes through the gizzard, where it is ground for digestion. And most chickens are raised in complete confinement, with inferior feed as their only source of food, suffering malnutrition of some degree, which results in fragile, brittle bones. Organic, free-range birds may be healthier themselves, but they are still delivering less-than-optimal nutrition and more-than-optimal saturated fat.

Check out how chicken stacks up to beef in nutrients, since everyone thinks chicken is healthier. Both contain 7 grams of protein per ounce. A skinless chicken breast has 0.9 grams of saturated fat in 3 ounces, while eye round steak has 1.4 grams of saturated fat. A skinless chicken thigh has 2.6 grams of saturated fat in 3 ounces and a tenderloin steak has 2.7 grams of saturated fat. Hey, what about that lower fat thing we thought we knew about chicken? It's time to rethink.

As for other fowl, we don't fare much better with them in our diet for similar reasons. High in fat, poorly nourished and raised in contaminated conditions, poultry just doesn't seem such a smart choice after all.

The Incredible Egg

Yes, eggs are a great source of protein. Yes, eggs are low in fat. Yes, a poached or hardboiled egg contains a mere 76 calories. But... one egg yolk contains 59 of those calories and more than two-thirds of your daily recommended cholesterol... one little yolk! That's a lot of cholesterol. There's more, though: Eggs are the seeds of their species—birds, reptiles or fish. Eggs symbolize the potential of an entire living, breathing creature. So in an egg, the character of a species is intensely concentrated. If you're wondering what that means to you, think about it. That one little egg is going to become a whole chicken. That's a lot of excess energy.

Now, while lots of different kinds of eggs are eaten by human beings, chicken eggs are, without question, the egg of choice in our culture. Considered to be one of the most versatile foods around, eggs have been removed from the "axis of evil" of foods and been restored to a place of honor and glory. But should they be? They have the unique ability to bind ingredients together, like in puddings, custards and sauces. They have an even more uncanny ability to expand and remain bound, like in meringue or cakes. Their shells are composed mostly of calcium carbonate and a bit of protein, with the yolk composed of water, fat and protein, as well as iron, cholesterol, lecithin and vitamin A. Egg whites are composed mostly of water and albumin (protein). So what about eggs? They have lots of energy in them; they bind and leaven, they have lots of protein and even calcium.

Eggs, by nature of their concentrated energy, cause the human body to contract. They give the body a very concentrated form of heat as our organs labor to break them down and assimilate them. Since they are one of the most concentrated forms of animal energy, eggs cause extreme reactions in us, like sweet cravings, the desire for hot spices and deep thirst—all attempts by the body to release and balance their intense drying energy. The strong binding nature of eggs as well as their ability to leaven cause the intestines to expand and contract with such intensity that digestion is greatly compromised.

Unlike other animal foods, eggs are generally free of antibiotics and growth hormones, making them less controversial than other choices. Should you decide that I'm a nice person and all—but nuts—and you are going to continue to eat some animal food, choose eggs. They are the least contaminated. Eggs from grass-fed birds are higher in folic acid, vitamin B_{12}, vitamin E and carotenes than cage-raised birds, so that's good. Some eggs are enriched with omega-3, an essential fatty acid, so that's good, too. There are organic eggs meaning that the farm has to allow the chickens to have access to outside areas during the day.

But before you run out to buy a dozen and tell all your friends that Christina said you can eat eggs; listen up: Most chickens are kept in cages, about five birds to a cage, each one with about half a square foot to move around in. That ain't much. On top of that, they have their beaks trimmed and in some cases their feet, so that they will not injure each other. Even the pope has been critical of keeping animals caged in this manner. The pope!

Okay, so you don't care that a chicken suffers to produce eggs. That's on you. But here's an interesting parting thought on eggs as far as women should be concerned. Traditionally seen as a symbol of fertility, an egg's twenty-one-day gestation period can definitely alter our natural twenty-eight-day cycle, throwing our natural clock into an imbalance, causing irregular menstruation and aggravated symptoms of PMS and menopause. Hot flashes have been shown to become much worse in women who eat eggs.

Nature's Perfect Food?

I think that dairy products should be illegal. They are, without question, the most lethal and unnatural food humans can consume.

We've been suckered by food marketers who promote dairy as the perfect food, with its high calcium and protein contents. Interestingly, nowadays many nutritionists and even more of the general public have begun to question the wisdom and safety of this food because they are coming to recognize that excessive consumption of dairy products has created human beings with deficient immune function, weak constitutions, brittle bones and rampant reproductive disorders. John McDougall, MD, author and nutrition expert, sees dairy products as the leading cause of allergies and has linked them with no fewer than forty-five diseases. Frank Oski, MD, author of *Don't Drink Your Milk* concurs, stating that milk so alters the human body that he would like to see it placed on an official hazardous food list. Finally, in her book *AIDS, Macrobiotics, and Natural Immunity*, Martha Cottrell, MD, cites major concerns with regards to dairy food consumption and immune function and degenerative disease The most recent studies conducted by Neal Barnard, MD, and T. Colin Campbell, MD, have shown results that should have us pouring this white poison down the drain by the gallon. Their work links dairy products to type 2 diabetes, digestive problems, prostate cancer and arthritis.

MOTHER'S MILK

I know that milk is our first food. It is the food that introduces us to the world outside of the womb. While it creates the bond between mother and child, it also prepares us for life away from her. It creates and nourishes us, reproducing within our species the patterns that make us human. Milk has the same job, species to species, to create and nourish the young of that species. And that's the key—to nourish the young of *that* species. When milk is consumed by the young of the same species, it imparts to them all of the characteristics, memories and behavior patterns of that species. To use the milk of one species to nourish another creates a tangled, confused identity crisis, to say the least.

Human beings are creatures of intuition, intelligence and creativity, with great capacity to think freely, and to act upon those thoughts. We are the only species (on earth, anyway) that can virtually create whatever it is that we envision, from bridges to technology to war. Drinking human mother's milk as our first food reinforces our human patterns, giving us the opportunity to be the best human we can be.

Now think about cow's milk, the most common choice for dairy food in our world. Cow's milk has the job to build cows. The rich, creamy textures of dairy foods are undoubtedly the basis of their appeal. They are also the same traits that create dependency—it's like you were never weaned. You are always at the breast. You grow dull with the consumption of dairy foods. Think about it: You break up with your lover and console yourselves with ice cream. Can't sleep? Try some warm milk; it'll knock you right out, dulled to the stress that might be keeping you awake. Dairy foods come from big, slow, dull, dependent animals—nice, cute, even, but dull as dust. Consuming great quantities of dairy may make you nice and passive, but not as sharp-witted and independent as humans have the potential to be.

Many of the current marketing concepts that call milk "the perfect food" are based on the fact that it contains all the vital nutrients essential to life. And that's true. Any mother creates the perfect food for her babies. Where it gets a little crazy is thinking that milk for cows, goats, rabbits, cats or even humans is the perfect food for any species other than their own.

Now, you can argue that humanity has used animal milk for centuries and that, of all species, humans have great capacity to consume anything. Both of these facts are true. There are even circumstances in life where the milk from another species can be used to effect a change in a condition. But we consume dairy foods—especially cow's milk—excessively, and therein is the harm.

So how did we get here? How did we get so dependent on the milk of cows? Even before we understood the makeup of cows' milk compared to humans', midwives for women who were having trouble nursing or if their milk would not come believed that cow's milk could serve humans. Infants took easily to the flavor, it was accessible and the infants appeared to thrive on it. And today, science appears to support the claim that cow's milk is a reasonable substitute. Human milk contains roughly 75 grams of lactose (a sugar in milk that is processed by your body to yield glucose for energy) for every quart of milk. Cow's milk has 45 grams of lactose per quart, which is the closest of any animal milk to human, at least as far as lactose is concerned.

However, the key to understanding why dairy products can prove more harmful than beneficial lies in understanding the role of *lactase* in the digestive process. We only hear about lactose and lactose intolerance, but lactase is critical. Lactase is an enzyme contained in the small intestine, with the job of breaking down the lactose in mother's milk. Lactase appears in an embryo's intestines during the last trimester, in preparation of digestion of mother's milk. Lactase naturally remains in the small intestine until the baby is about a year old. It begins to wane then, although it can remain relatively active up to about four years old. With the dwindling production of lactase, our ability to digest lactose also dwindles. Here's the interesting part: If the amount of lactose present in the intestines is more than the lactase needed for digestion, the lactose accumulates undigested in the large intestine where it ferments in the natural heat of the body, causing various chemical reactions with the bacteria that reside there. Eventually it turns into carbon dioxide and lactic acid, which together cause water retention in body tissue. You have just created a lactose-intolerant condition.

The protein in milk, *casein* (sodium caseinate), is really tough to digest. A very sticky protein, most of casein goes undigested in the body, and instead accumulates in soft tissue, causing sluggish circulation and inhibited digestion. Because casein is soft and dense, it's not the best protein for building and strengthening muscle tissue, which, in case you forgot, is the main reason we need protein in our bodies in the first place. Casein also has the unique ability to bind—so much so that it's an ingredient in some plastic and glue products…yummy. What that means is that as this protein is moving around inside a body that cannot digest it (at least most of the time), it will pull together and eventually form fatty cysts and tumors.

MORE BAD NEWS ABOUT DAIRY FAT

The fat in dairy products is even more fun for our health and waistline than the protein. Saturated fats (the fat from dairy foods) will accumulate in the body, causing a hardened, bulky layer over our muscles, will slow metabolism so we get nice and fat (think cow) and will inhibit oxygen getting to body tissue. It means we won't use oxygen well and with the degeneration of tissue, we grow lethargic and depressed.

Fat-free dairy foods aren't the answer, though. Skim milk, fat-free and low-fat milk are all by-products of whole milk. All that's removed is the fat. It really doesn't improve the milk or its effect on us—it still contains both casein and lactose. It actually concentrates the protein, which leads us to the Holy Grail of dairy, calcium.

BUILDS STRONG BONES...

Milk is loaded with calcium. We know this because advertising tells us it's true. Just about every celebrity with a face has posed for those ads with a milk mustache telling us that milk has lots of calcium and is good for us. (I question the wisdom of using sports celebrities, models and TV stars as nutrition experts, but that's me.) What no one tells you is this: Calcium is bonded to casein. And since your body has so much trouble digesting casein, that should tell us something about the usability of dairy calcium.

Just because dairy has calcium doesn't mean your body benefits. I guess the milk marketers aren't detail-oriented...so they forget little words like *digestible*. We can utilize only about 12% of the calcium in dairy, leaving most of it undigested in the body. Without magnesium or phosphorous, we can't digest calcium, and neither of these elements are in dairy foods unless they are enriched.

Did you know that most of the people in the world don't rely on dairy foods for their calcium? Or that Americans take in twice the amount of dairy as most of the world? Protein-rich diets, like those of people consuming great amounts of dairy, produce a greater excretion of urea (or blood urea nitrogen) from the kidneys, depleting the body of essential nutrients like calcium, magnesium and potassium. It's interesting to note that the incidence of osteoporosis is significantly higher among people who consume great quantities of animal protein. For example, Eskimos, who consume tremendous amounts of protein and calcium, have the highest incidence of osteoporosis in the world. In contrast, among many African peoples who exist on low-protein, low-calcium diets, osteoporosis is extremely rare, if not totally absent.

There's more. Your body loves balance and will strive for it, with or without your help. Poor digestion of casein and lactose and the intake of high-concentrated protein from fat-free dairy foods cause the blood to become highly acidic. Can you guess what the body relies on to counter an overly acidic condition? It's calcium that dissolves in the blood (known as serum calcium).

The use of dairy for calcium not only causes the body to accumulate unusable calcium, it makes the body require more calcium. And metabolism slows, since serum calcium is essential to that function. As we eat more dairy products, the cycle continues.

Your best bet is to choose vegetables and beans that are rich in useable calcium: dark leafy greens, black beans, soy products, whole grains and sea plants. And by reducing the amount of animal protein in your diet, your need for calcium is also reduced, since you will lose less in the digestive process. You can get all the calcium you need from the food you eat, if you choose wisely. And supplements? For certain conditions, like preexisting osteopenia and osteoporosis, of course, supplementing calcium is much needed to stabilize the condition. Again, don't play Marcus Welby; see your doctor before popping pills.

Say Cheese

Cheese, which is considered by many to be the food of the gods, is anything but. Cheese is made by acidifying milk, adding bacteria and enzymes (rennet) to convert the casein (milk protein) from soluble to insoluble so the milk will jell. The lactose converts to simple sugar. Enzymes coagulate the casein; whey is pressed and the fat, protein and lactose are broken into simple molecules by bacteria, resulting in cheese—a very concentrated and solid form of dairy protein and fat. The production of most cheese relies heavily on various molds and bacteria, which can wreak havoc on your digestive tract, resulting in bloating and the accumulation of mucus in your intestines. Cheese causes the body to become acidic, resulting in damp intestines, pale skin, fluid retention, kidney stones and wrinkles.

One last point: Cheese is so calorically dense that it can double the calories in a recipe. Yikes!

Three Main Ingredients of French Cooking: Butter, Butter and . . . Butter?

Ah, French food: decadent, rich, creamy, buttery dishes that can send you into fits of orgasmic delight—and your heart into fits of angina. While most

French chefs in America would have us believe that butter must be the base of just about every dish worth eating, the truth is that butter is brutal for your overall health and weight.

Interestingly, in France, butter is used far more sparingly than in "French" cooking in America. Their overall portions are smaller; they drink a bit of red wine, which helps the body to digest fat; and they eat a lot of vegetables. (They probably get more daily exercise than the average American, too, even though they may not be considered a "fitness" culture.)

Butter is made by agitating cream until granules form and bond. This dense, fatty substance is about 80% fat. While butter is high in short-chain fatty acids, these are not fatty acids the human body needs, and can even inhibit our own metabolism of essential fatty acids.

Butter is a stable fat for cooking, with the ability to remain so under heat. This should tell you something—like how hard it is to break down in the heat of our intestines as we attempt to digest it. Instead of stable fat, perhaps we should think of butter as accumulating fat…on our hips, thighs, bellies, around our hearts, in our veins and arteries. Yum!

We All Scream for Ice Cream

Ice cream, my personal favorite—at least it was when I was growing up. The effects of the dense protein and fats of dairy food are, in essence, concentrated in ice cream. Combining them with sugar and freezing temperatures make ice cream as indigestible as a dairy food can get. Anything that is freezing cold will cause organ function to slow, growing sluggish, accumulating fat, especially in the intestines. As congestion builds in the digestive tract, it is more difficult to oxygenate the brain, and we begin to feel dull. Think about the times in life when ice cream has tasted best to you. This frozen, sweet food is great for numbing body function and for paralyzing us emotionally.

But wait! What about all this recent hoo-ha about dairy helping us to lose weight? Isn't it worth the health risk if you can be thinner? A large study conducted by *Pediatrics* on 12,000 children nationwide found that those who drank three or more servings of milk a day gained weight. And the more milk they drank, the more weight they gained. Oops. And then there's Michael Zemel, a nutrition professor at University of Tennessee whose study results were the driving force behind the Three-a-Day campaign designed to convince people that milk made you skinny. Basing his claims on a study done on obese African-Americans, he came to the conclusion that calcium in milk was the reason for the weight loss. But let's let the facts speak here. In a study published in the *Journal of the American College of Nutrition* (vol. 26, no. 5), fifty-eight premenopausal women (divided into three groups) were given calcium supplements, low-fat milk or a placebo for twelve weeks as a part of a reduced-calorie diet and regular exercise program. Neither of the groups taking supplements or low-fat milk showed acceleration in weight loss. According to the *Journal*, Zemel's was the third study of its kind to show similar results. All the women in this particular study group showed significant weight and body fat loss, but they also were adhering to an exercise program and reducing their caloric intake. Duh!

So how did Zemel come to his conclusions? The general consensus is that the study used people who ate a very low-calcium diet and when their calcium intake increased, they lost weight, as they would. If you read the fine print of the studies, you will see successful weight loss statistics, but it is unlikely that it is due to dairy consumption. The study states that consuming dairy, along with a reduced-calorie diet plan, will result in weight loss. But is it due to the dairy intake or the reduced-calorie diet? The study reveals that the participants lost about one pound per week on a high-dairy diet. These same participants reduced their caloric intake by five hundred calories a day. In any diet plan, reducing your intake by five hundred calories a day will result in losing about one pound per week. Zemel's study was done on thirty people, five of them men—and only eleven of them were on the high-dairy diet. Not exactly a real-world sample group. With the Dairy Council spending more than $200 million since 2003 marketing this weight-loss claim and Zemel holding a highly unusual patent on said claim, it has to make you wonder about the authenticity.

The bottom line is that while many studies on dairy and weight gain are inconclusive, several have shown a positive link between dairy food consumption and obesity. Some researchers say that calcium helps to promote weight loss, but most agree that the hormones, whey protein and milk fat are likely contributors to obesity. That's enough for me.

HOW SWEET IT IS!

Sugar, whether it's organic, raw, unrefined or the common white table version will make you fat and unhealthy. But fighting a sweet tooth can be an uphill battle—one that you'd like to win by weaning yourself off sweets.

And that's hard. But artificial sweeteners are not the answer to your sugar-plum dreams either. These products, marketed as a dieter's dream, can easily become your worst nightmare. They are synthesized chemicals—and you know much your liver just loves those, don't you? Artificial sweeteners interrupt the liver's ability to regulate your metabolism, and a balanced metabolism is essential to achieving your ideal weight. And, not to put too fine a point on it, but because they interrupt your body's natural calorie gauge, you will actually eat more food.

So how did we become so enslaved to these toxic treats? Simple. Desperation and marketing are the perfect marriage. People love sweet taste and marketers know this. So they fill your head with the nonsense that if you use these sugar substitutes, you can have your cake and eat it, too. Well, considering that we are now a nation that seems as addicted to artificial sweeteners as we are to the "real" thing and are still struggling with ever-increasing waistlines, I think we can agree that those little pink, blue and yellow packets may not be the answer.

Let's look at these insidious sweeteners and their impact on your health (besides contributing to making you fat).

"A" is for *aspartame*, known in natural circles as sweet poison. A non-saccharide sweetener, aspartame is most often used in beverages, as it is unstable under heat and loses much of its sweetness in cooking. Upon ingestion, aspartame breaks down into several chemicals, including formaldehyde. Associated with more than ninety-two different health side effects, this chemical dissolves into a solution that makes its way through your body and can settle in any tissue, anywhere. Aspartame does not break down in the human body and dissolve.

And how do you know if it is affecting your health? Check out some of these symptoms and see if they fit you: decreased vision, pain in your eyes, trouble with contact lenses, decreased tear production, ringing in your ears, sensitivity to noise, headaches, migraines, dizziness, restless legs, memory loss, hyperactivity, irritability, insomnia, depression, shortness of breath, abdominal pain, painful swallowing, loss of control of diabetes, sudden weight gain, severe PMS. Gee, don't we medicate for a lot of these? Maybe you need to just quit using aspartame-sweetened products instead. Sure, your symptoms can be the result of other things, but isn't it funny that all of these ailments can be linked to this artificial sweetener that is so prevalent in our food? It sure is worth considering.

Of course, you could switch to Sweet 'N Low and get a daily dose of saccharin to can increase your risk of bladder tumors, among other things. The oldest artificial sweetener, saccharin is different than aspartame, although lethal in its own way to your health. Made from benzoic sulfinide, saccharin has no food energy and is stable under heat. It doesn't react chemically with other foods (unlike aspartame) and stores well. In its day, saccharin was important because it went right through the human digestive system without being digested. Investigations of this sweetener began with Teddy Roosevelt's administration and continue to this day, with the risks of bladder and other cancers hanging over it like a specter.

But the mother of all artificial sweeteners, the queen of the chemical table, the winner of the hearts and minds of Americans everywhere is *sucralose*, marketed under the brand name Splenda. Even the name is seductive. And the marketing is pure genius. What could be so bad? It's just like sugar, because it's made from sugar…and sugar's natural, right?

Well, Grasshopper, here's a little reality check: Despite the dusting of calorie-free pixie dust in the commercials, Splenda is a health nightmare just waiting to happen. Currently the number one artificial sweetener, this toxic sweetener can be found in more than 3,500 products on your grocer's shelves.

But it's made from sugar, right? Well, to be truthful, there is a shred of truth to this claim. Splenda does start off as a sugar molecule, but that is where the similarities end. Once the end product emerges from the patented five-step process, it bears absolutely no resemblance to what people recognize as sugar.

Even a quick trip to the Splenda website and you will see that it is not natural and certainly is no longer sugar. So what is it? Plainly stated, Splenda is a synthesized chemical. Sounds yummy. Three hydroxyl groups of atoms are removed from a molecule of sugar and replaced with three atoms of chlorine. According the Marion Nestle, PhD, the chlorine makes the sweetener unavailable to digestive enzymes, meaning that you excrete it intact and, hence, no calories. And by the time the processing of Splenda is complete, the original sugar molecule has become a chlorocarbon, a highly toxic compound that has no place in the human body.

The manufacturer of Splenda claims that extensive safety studies have been conducted. However, most of the studies to get manufacturing approval were done on lab rats, mice, rabbits and guinea pigs. Don't even get me started on animal testing. It's cruel, devastating to the animals and, in the end, has little to do with how a product will behave in humans.

Splenda is touted as having no calories per serving, and in this age of epidemic obesity, that is considered a good thing. Actually, it has 96 calories in a cup, much less than sugar, but the cost to your health can be higher than can be measured in pounds.

The whole artificial sweetener thing is just plain crazy. If you are under the impression that anything in those little packets is remotely natural or good for your health, think again.

SOME REAL SWEET NEWS

So are you doomed to a life that lacks sweet taste? Is there no dessert in your future if you are to maintain a healthy weight and keep your body vital and strong? There are so many options that are natural and are good for you. Some, admittedly, have more calories than you might like while trying to drop a few pounds, but I'll show you some low- and no-calorie options, with no chlorine-sprinkling fairies to be seen!

I use *agave nectar, brown rice syrup* and *barley malt* in my own cooking, as they are natural and made from complex carbohydrates. They do have calories, so they do not give you a free pass to live on desserts. Trust me on that one; that's where I went astray... big-time!

Agave is made from cactus plants and is slowly absorbed by the body, so there are no sugar rushes with this delicate sweetener. It is about 75% sweeter than sugar, so you should taste the agave in its raw state before using it so you can gauge the level of flavor you want.

Brown rice syrup and barley malt, which are made from fermented whole grains, also digest slowly and have great flavor. Brown rice syrup is about half as sweet as sugar, so play with it to get the sweet level you desire. I love its delicate sweetness and it remains high on my list of sweet choices. Barley malt has a flavor reminiscent of molasses, so be sure you that's the taste you're looking for in your dessert before using it.

All three of these healthy options have 20 to 23 calories per teaspoon, which is very close to sugar, but they are much healthier for you in the long run as they are complex carbohydrate sweeteners and will not spike your blood sugar. But you can't use them freely, unless you want to carry around a bit of excess you. It takes a bit of practice to use them in cooking. They are liquid sweeteners with the texture of honey, so you must adjust your batter and dough recipes to accommodate that extra fluid. But it's easy once you experiment a little.

Date sugar, maple syrup, organic cane juice (organic sugar) and *turbinado sugar* are all healthier options than refined white sugar, but in my view, not by much. They are calorically dense simple sugars, so they land you on that roller coaster of ups and downs with your energy. They suppress immune function, so they make you tired. I say skip them. And since most of these options to sugar or artificial sweeteners are very close in calorie content to sugar, why not choose the healthiest option?

Honey is in a class by itself. A simple sugar, honey is calorically dense, so it can make you fat if eaten in excess. But honey is different than other mono-saccharides in that it is an inverted sugar, meaning that it digests slowly and doesn't send your glucose levels off the charts, like other simple sugars. On top of that, honey is rich in antioxidants and is a great source for digestible iron, so it can make your red blood quite strong, which is good. Just take care with this sweetener; it can pack on the pounds. And for the purest of pure vegans out there, I will tell you that I do not consider honey to be an animal product. In the local hives I have visited, where I purchase my organic raw honey, the bees are treated like royalty, so I have made my peace with my choice. It is not my first choice of sweeteners, but I would be remiss in skipping over it.

No-Cal and All-Natural

But I did promise you no-calorie, natural options for sweet taste, didn't I? Well, there are two that I think are worth mentioning here. The first, *stevia*, is a concentrate made from an herb and is usually available in powder or liquid form. This intensely sweet herb is said to be a natural substitute for sugar. With a concentrated sweet flavor—1 teaspoon is equal to 2 cups of sugar or 200 to 300 times sweeter than sugar. This one is a bit cloying for me; overwhelming, in fact. Many people swear by it and couldn't live without it. If you like it, there's no bad news, so have at it. You can cook and bake with it, but the results can be intensely sweet, as the flavor concentrates as it cooks. Have fun with it and see how it goes for you.

My newest favorite sweetener is called *erythritol*. Don't panic; it sounds like a chemical, but it's as natural as sugar. In fact, it is fermented sugar alcohol, so it comes from sugar. The natural process doesn't upset your tummy, is about 70 to 80% as sweet as sugar, works like sugar, is granular like sugar, does not promote cavities in your teeth and seems to be safe even for diabetics. And since your intestines don't absorb it, it has no calories…none. I love the flavor of this one and there seems to be no bad news here either. It has a delicate sweetness and fine granules, which blend well in recipes.

Maybe you *can* have your cake and eat it…

EAT MORE, LOSE MORE

You know that eating vegetables has lots of health benefits. (You do know that, right?) While it just makes common sense to eat them, vegetables can actually be a key factor in you finding your way to your ideal weight—deliciously.

Naturally low in fat and calories, vegetables are rich sources of dietary fiber, making them the trifecta of weight loss. Since they are low in calories, you can eat a lot of them and enjoy a ton of energy. But the news gets even better. The high-fiber content of vegetables fills your tummy faster and keeps you full longer, so no more bingeing! But here is the real kicker: Vegetables provide the body with many essential nutrients that create the energy to fuel muscle cells. This gives you energy to burn, which makes you feel more vital, which creates a desire to be active, which in turns burns calories. Getting the picture here?

Vegetables are even low in sodium; and while you may be wondering about the importance of that little fact, consider this. The average person carries around about five pounds of extra weight as a result of sodium consumption, which causes the intestines to hold fluid. Eating less sodium will allow your body to release that excess fluid. You can practically feel that flat stomach already, can't you?

BEST VEG FOR WEIGHT LOSS

So are there vegetables that are better for weight loss than others? Yup. Contrary to what a lot of proponents of high-protein diets would have you believe, most vegetables will not contribute to your weight problem. You did not get fat from eating carrots. In fact, there are some veggies that can really help you in your bid to lose some excess you and can kick-start the process of fat burning, keep you sated and be valuable tools in your weight-loss program.

THE ROOT OF THE SOLUTION

Of course, it makes sense that sweeter, starchier vegetables are a bit more calorically dense than other veggies. Winter squash, carrots, parsnips, sweet potatoes, beets and potatoes are all in that category. So should you eat less of them to lose some pounds? Most people screw up their weight-loss plans with sweets. The lack of sweet comfort in many weight-loss plans can really sabotage the best intentions. When the decadent sugary seduction of a brownie has you in its grip, a bowl of steamed kale, even with balsamic vinegar on it, will hardly break the chokehold. On the other hand, if your body is used to eating carrots, winter squash and sweet potatoes in small quantities but on a regular basis, then the grip of sugar is loosened on you. You don't crave sweets as much because your body is getting that comforting taste all the time.

From the perspective of Chinese medicine (of which I am a proponent if you haven't figured that out) the spleen, pancreas and stomach are all connected and are said to create our center of stability, perseverance and resourcefulness—all valuable traits in the quest for health and ideal weight.

Mild, sweet taste (not sugar sweet but the natural sweet of vegetables) is the flavor that animates and strengthens these organs, allowing them to do their jobs efficiently; sweet foods relax the body and settle us comfortably. When your blood sugar is stable, so are you. Keeping these three organs in balance helps us to maintain our sense of direction in life, sure of our abilities and conscious of how deep our capacities run. We live in a culture powered by sugar and I think we can agree that generally we lack the focus of a heat-seeking missile. (Is there anybody who doesn't know what ADD stands for?) When your body is overrun with sugar and your blood chemistry is in chaos, you have no energy to commit to the challenge of making your dreams a reality. When we are overcome with sugar and artificial sweeteners, we can't cope with challenges or adversities, let alone have discipline. Believe me; losing weight and keeping it off (without a change in thinking) is demanding and requires some discipline.

When we eat sugar as a food group, we tend to have loose, weak muscles, especially in the legs. Women will tend to hold weight in the lower body, bulking up in the buttocks and thighs. Men will hold the weight in their midsection, looking soft and doughy. Interestingly, the loose muscle tone will show strongly in the face, too, with ill-defined features and slack facial expressions. It looks as though you have no definition, slightly puffy without sharp, clear expression, with washed-out color.

What does this have to do with winter squash? The spleen, pancreas and stomach serve as the storage organs for the blood supply to the body as it requires. They also serve as an integral part of the lymphatic system, protecting the body from infection. The spleen also serves as the organ that holds elements that are taken from damaged cells, again, for use later when the body needs them. Note that all these functions have to do with the gathering of resources, storage for us to draw upon as the needs arise.

The pancreas has the job of regulating our blood sugar levels, which is our body's way of controlling our stored resources of energy. If it's overworked it becomes aggravated and depleted and alters how our body functions.

Here's the connection. Since we, as human beings, have a conscious connection to our body and how we feel, we are aware of our resources and how full or low our stores are. Look at hypoglycemia as an example. As a culture, we consume tremendous amounts of simple, refined sugars, which break down very quickly and enter the bloodstream almost upon consumption, instantly altering the blood chemistry. As a result, blood sugar levels are all over the place, rising and dropping dramatically, creating extremes from high levels of nervous energy to lethargy and weakness. As your blood sugar drops and you have no reserves to draw upon, you grow weak, with trembling limbs and, in more serious cases, disorientation. Your solution? You take in more sugar—candy, chocolate, cookies, orange juice—to quickly raise your blood sugar to a more normal level and your body back to functioning. The problem is that with simple sugars, you are not creating any stores of energy for the body to draw on to keep the blood sugar levels on an even keel. As you continue this pattern, the dramatic shifts in blood sugar levels weaken the organs, especially the pancreas. You will find that the elated feelings of energy that you get from sugar grow shorter and shorter, requiring more and more sugar to create normal function. You take in more and more empty calories, increasing the size of your waistline and your risk of diabetes.

So what do we do? Vegetables that grow close to the ground, with sweet flavor as their signature: winter squash (including butternut, buttercup, acorn, Hubbard, pumpkin, Hokkaido), artichokes, carrot, parsnip and beets will serve you well to balance blood sugar, hold sugar cravings at bay and help you get your weight under control. So before you turn your back on the starchy, sweet vegetables that you may have come to fear, try a little experiment. Include modest amounts of those vegetables in your daily diet for seven to ten days and see how your sweet cravings loosen their grip on you. Just don't cook them with butter, brown sugar and marshmallows. Gotcha!

Skinny Greens for Skinny Jeans

Leafy greens, in particular bitter greens, can be one of your best choices to get the process of weight loss started. In Chinese medicine, it is held that bitter and sour flavor animates and supports the function of your liver. Remember that your largest gland has the essential job of supporting your body in the metabolism of your macronutrients, known to you as fat, protein and carbohydrates. So it just makes sense that if your liver is working well, doing its job efficiently and at its peak, your body can assimilate nutrients in the best way that your body can use them and not store them as excess. Your liver also has the job of aiding your body in ridding itself of toxins. For a little gland, it has some seriously important jobs to do. Your liver function determines whether or not you can stabilize your weight. But the liver has no idea how to handle artificial chemicals. They are completely foreign to our internal environment. So when your liver is constantly bombarded by these compounds, it works overtime to do all the jobs required of it as well as trying to get rid of these toxins.

High-fructose corn syrup, chemical additives, preservatives, pesticides, herbicides, fungicides, artificial colorings, sucralose, artificial sweeteners and foods that are chemically enriched—all these toxins bombard your liver every single hour of every single day if you are eating a typical American diet. Your liver is exhausted trying to metabolize nutrients, usually way more than you need. Your liver has to try and figure out what to do with all those nutrients, deciphering between the empty calories and the valuable ones, and then you hit it right between the eyes with poisonous compounds that it can't process. And you wonder why you can't lose weight without a major, permanent shift in your food choices?

Dark, leafy, bitter greens—like broccoli rabe, escarole, watercress, arugula, baby spinach, dandelion and mustard greens—work to aid your exhausted liver, breaking down fat and protein, creating a drier liver environment through their astringent nature. These greens, along with foods like barley, oats, lemons, limes and good-quality vinegars can be invaluable tools in rebalancing your liver so it can do the job it was meant to do— metabolize your nutrients so you can draw on them to create the energy you need to be active.

DIET SPECIALISTS IN THE VEGETABLE WORLD

There are also some vegetables that I think of as "diet specialists." They are like your own little secret weapons in the battle of the bulge. My favorites are daikon and shiitake and maitake mushrooms. These humble veggies will change your life!

Daikon is a long, elegant white root, also known as the icicle or Satsuma radish and has been prized in Asia for centuries for what it can do for human health. In Chinese medicine, we say that daikon helps to kickstart the weight-loss process because it has an astringent nature that aids the liver in metabolism of fat and protein. If you have eaten in a Japanese restaurant and enjoyed some tempura, you will have noticed that a small dish of a liquidy white ingredient comes with it. When you bite into it, a hot peppery flavor explodes on your tongue. Japanese chefs know that a small amount of grated fresh daikon will help you to digest the oil in the tempura. But don't even consider taking a baggie of grated daikon with you to the mall for your fried onion-ring binge! For the occasional deep-fried side dish, grated daikon can be your best pal in digesting.

All that sounds good, but if it's cold, hard facts that you want, here they are. The best vitamins and minerals to stimulate weight loss include riboflavin (for normal thyroid function), niacin (part of the glucose tolerance factor that releases every time blood sugar rises), pantothenic acid (assists in energy production and adrenal function), vitamin B_6 (essential to thyroid hormone production and metabolism), choline (not really a vitamin, but a compound made in the liver that's responsible for fat metabolism), vitamin C (aids in the conversion of glucose to energy in our cells), chromium (a mineral required for the metabolism of sugar), manganese (which also helps regulate the metabolism of sugar) and zinc (which helps regulate appetite and the release of insulin). Where do you get all these valuable tools for weight loss? Every single one of them exists in substantial quantities in daikon. Its unique combination of nutrients makes daikon one of your best assets in achieving your ideal weight.

Daikon's delicate, peppery flavor makes it an absolute pleasure to eat as well. From salads to stews, casseroles and oven-roasted dishes, its distinct flavor makes it the perfect accompaniment to any other veggie. Its clean taste supports the characters around it, making sweet taste sweeter, sour a little more so and spicy flavor develops just a touch more nuance. It's pretty amazing.

The most effective way to use daikon in weight loss is in soup. With hot broth as the vehicle, its nutrients get delivered to the cells more efficiently. The power of daikon goes to work more quickly and effectively. So a lovely veggie soup with daikon in the cast of characters a couple of times a week will be just what your waistline ordered!

And did I mention that daikon is also a rich source of cancer-fighting compounds?

Shiitake mushrooms are one of those crazy foods that people have heard about but have no idea of the power contained within these humble fungi. We often classify them as vegetables, because *fungus* sounds so unappealing. But all mushrooms belong to the fungi family and are not the same as the fungus you may be thinking about.

Once again, Asian wisdom trumps the West with shiitakes. Used for more than six thousand years, shiitakes are said to be the key to longevity and maintenance of a healthy weight. Their smoky flavor has caught on in the United States but it wasn't the taste that brought them to the attention of the Chinese. Chinese medicine says that eating shiitake mushrooms cleanses the blood and boosts immune function. Shiitakes contain lentinan, a polysaccharide shown to have active anticancer capacity and to be a powerful immune booster. Many studies have since shown the effectiveness of lentinan to diminish and "starve" tumors.

But here's where shiitakes first got our attention here in America. The spores in the shiitake contain a compound called eritadenine. Who? With heart disease as the primary cause of death in this country for both men and women, you might want to remember this word because this compound lowers cholesterol levels—and it lowers them regardless of the dietary fats being eaten. Shiitake mushrooms can reduce blood pressure and lower cholesterol in numbers unmatched by any pharmaceutical. Interestingly, the more regularly you eat them, the more your levels drop.

My stepmother was really struggling with her cholesterol numbers and hated the idea of changing her very Irish diet of meat and potatoes all round, with an egg thrown in for variety. I finally convinced her to add a shiitake mushroom to her beef stew or chicken soup twice a week. In just four months, she showed a drop of more than fifty points in her levels of LDL, the "bad" cholesterol. She was so impressed that she did in fact, change her diet and became a quasi-vegetarian. (Well, we all have to start somewhere.)

But what does this antioxidant-rich, fiber-loaded mushroom have to do with weight loss? Acting as a blood cleanser, shiitakes work as a support system for your liver in its job of metabolizing your macronutrients. With pantothenic acid, vitamin C, manganese and selenium as a part of their nutritional profile, shiitakes work in the body to "soften" hardened accumulations of fat, which your body can then discharge. And when your body dumps fat, you can lose weight. See?

Available dried or fresh, shiitakes should have a regular place on your table. The dried versions require reconstitution by soaking in cold water until tender, but the drying process intensifies their power, so I tend to use the dried when I need their "medicine," if you get my drift. Fresh shiitakes are milder in flavor and very soft so they cook quickly, but they're no nutritional wimps. So whichever shiitake you can find, use them once or twice a week in soups, sauces and stir-fry dishes.

Along with shiitake, a new player in the weight-loss arena is maitake mushrooms. Known as the "dancing mushroom" because foragers danced with joy when they found these prized fungi, research now shows that maitake do more than inspire spontaneous soft-shoe routines.

The active ingredients in maitake responsible for its newfound fame are polysachharides called "beta-glucans." Maitakes contain a unique beta-glucan called "D-fraction," which may be responsible for many of its health benefits. Much of the research being done on maitakes places the focus on cancer prevention and treatment, specifically the inhibition of tumor growth. There is also growing acceptance of eating maitakes during chemotherapy; they are so effective in boosting the immune system that they can make treatments easier to endure.

The newest research also shows that maitake mushrooms can help you reduce an expanding waistline. Low in calories, maitakes are packed with a lot of vitamins and minerals. But here's where the beta-glucan D-fraction comes in to play. According to PETA's website, in a study done in Japan, thirty overweight participants took a supplement of maitake and made no other dietary or lifestyle changes—not one, nada. After eight weeks, each patient had lost eleven to thirteen pounds, with some losing twenty-five pounds! What makes these results amazing is the short timeframe of the study and the fact that the participants made no other changes.

Imagine what your results would be if you made changes to the way you eat, added exercise to your life, and ate maitakes in soup once or twice a week?

How Much Is Enough—Even of a Good Thing

Okay, so you're now hip to the idea of eating your veggies on a daily basis. How much do you need to see the benefits of these glorious foods? That would be eight to ten servings a day. What?!?!?! It sounds like a lot, so let me make sense of it for you. A serving of vegetables, by conventional nutrition standards would look like one of these: ½ cup of chopped vegetables, 1 cup raw salad greens, six to eight 3-inch carrot sticks, 1 medium sweet potato or ¾ cup vegetable juice. Go grab a measuring cup and some veggies from your well-stocked fridge (I can dream, can't I?). Measure out ½ cup of chopped vegetables, 1 cup of salad greens, lay a potato on the plate and pour a lovely glass of V-8 or other veggie juice. Add some protein and you have a meal that has four of your needed servings at one sitting. Make a bowl of vegetable soup. Eat that with a salad, a whole grain and some protein and wow…you've done it again. Eat two meals a day that look like this (not counting your two snacks) and you get eight servings without breaking a sweat! And I haven't even figured fruit into the mix. Just 1 medium apple or pear, ½ cup of berries, a dozen grapes or ½ grapefruit makes a serving. Notice that the fruit servings are smaller. With more sugar, fruit has more calories and has to be eaten with a bit more care when trying to lose weight. Sure it's better than a Snickers bar, but not as good as carrots or broccoli.

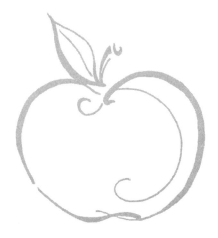

5

Eat Well for Life

Knowledge must come through action; you can have no
test which is not fanciful, save by trial.   —SOPHOCLES

I'm always fascinated by the diet crazes that continue to sweep the
nation. *Craze* is the operative word for me. Each one seems nuttier than
the one that precedes it. Why do we fall for them? We want desperately
to lose weight, but we seem to think that we can do it with no effort, sac-
rifice or change to our lifestyle and eating habits. We buy book after book;
watch show after show, hoping that one of these approaches will be the one
to do the job. When will we stop being fools? Education followed by action
is the key to success, just like anything else. You really can't continue to "eat
the foods you love" and lose weight for life. I don't care what Jenny says.

The first known diet book was published in 1864 by an English casket-
maker, William Banting. He needed a change because he could no longer
tie his shoes and had gotten so fat he had to walk down the stairs backward. His book, *Letter of Corpulence*, called for low-carbohydrate foods and
a daily portion of alcohol. It sold 58,000 copies. Not much else was published until 1961, when Herman Taller wrote *Calories Don't Count*, which
linked the intake of simple carbohydrates and sugar to obesity. It sold
2 million copies. Then in 1967, Irwin Stillman published *The Quick Weight-
Loss Diet* and sold 20 million copies of a high-protein, low-carbohydrate
diet. In 1972, Robert Atkins published his first version of the high-protein,

low-carbohydrate diet, *The Diet Revolution*. Diet history was made. In 1978, *The Scarsdale Diet* became a national bestseller, advocating a seven-hundred-calorie a day, high-protein diet. In 1992, Dr. Atkins reissued his book as *The New Diet Revolution*, again a bestseller and the most popular of these diet plans. Since then diet books have flooded the shelves of bookstores everywhere, with no end in sight. And America just gets fatter.

So what's up with diets and the thinking that is behind them?

High-Protein Diets

Diet gurus, even some with impressive medical degrees behind their names, who tout the glories of high-protein and fat-laden diets continue to grab the attention of millions of desperate dieters. The truth about these types of fad diets is that people can temporarily lose large amounts of weight and can even lower their blood cholesterol, sugar and triglycerides—but not in a healthy and sustainable way.

The foods recommended for a high-protein diet are mainly meat, egg and dairy products (which are high in cholesterol), fat and animal protein. (See chapter 4.) These foods are deficient in dietary fiber and carbohydrates; are often contaminated with chemicals and microbes; and are imbalanced when it comes to vitamins and minerals. Sure, there are some veggies in these diet plans as well, but wow, a lot of meat! Recommendations to eat fewer animal products and more plant foods have been made by just about every health organization, from the American Heart Association to the American Cancer Society and all the professional and medical groups in between. All of these respected organizations agree that many of the chronic illnesses plaguing modern Western society are caused by an unhealthy diet and lifestyle, including a lack of exercise. Improving and maintaining good health and managing your weight comes from eating fewer animal products and a more plant food–based diet. But yet high-protein diets continue to thrive among those trying to lose weight.

Meats, eggs, poultry and dairy products have been directly linked to most cases of obesity; cardiovascular diseases; adult-onset diabetes; breast, colon and prostate cancer, gallbladder disease; kidney failure; multiple sclerosis; rheumatoid arthritis; constipation; diverticulosis; hemorrhoids and hiatal hernia. Whew! You don't have to be a rocket scientist to see that the risk of becoming sick increases with your intake of these foods.

And did I mention your bones? Among other things, high-protein diets cause serious metabolic changes that lead to bone loss and kidney stones. Red meat, poultry, fish, shellfish and eggs tend to be more acidic in structure. By nature, plant foods are alkaline in our bodies. Our bodies fiercely guard their acid-alkaline balance (pH), so all of our pH-driven biochemical functions take place smoothly. The acid overload that results from high-protein animal foods must be somehow buffered. And interestingly, that primary buffer comes from your bones. They literally dissolve into phosphates and calcium for just this purpose. This is the first step in the loss of bone density, which leads to osteoporosis. The second step consists of altered kidney physiology that increases the acid load, resulting in the loss of substantial quantities of bone material, including calcium into the urine. And the presence of this bone material in our kidneys also lays the foundation for calcium-based kidney stones.

Just to clarify, there are two basic high-protein approaches: the ones that limit calorie intake to induce a state known as "ketosis," limiting or eliminating carbohydrate consumption, and ones that impose stringent rules that limit the your intake of food across the board, from every food group.

The first style, "a ketogenic diet," is the approach taken by Dr. Atkins. This kind of diet causes your body to produce ketones (acidic byproducts of metabolism), by severely restricting the intake of carbohydrates. At the same time, a high consumption of fat and protein is allowed. With this type of diet, there is an insufficient amount of your body's primary fuel, carbohydrate. Your body turns to the fat from food, as well as body fat for use as fuel. The resulting condition, ketosis, is a toxic state associated with loss of appetite, nausea, fatigue, low blood pressure—and weight loss. By eliminating most, if not all carbohydrates from your diet, along with a suppressed appetite, the obvious result is a decrease in caloric intake. Therefore, ketosis is the key to the diet's success: Your body starves but you don't suffer hunger pangs. (Remember that protein is very filling and your appetite is suppressed.) By the way, ketosis also occurs naturally when people are starving to death or seriously ill. Add to that the fact that this diet is made up of the foods that most nutrition experts tell us contribute dramatically to our most common causes of death and disability—meat, eggs, poultry, dairy and the saturated fats that come along with them, and what you have is a recipe for health disaster.

So why then did this method of dieting become so popular? Because you can drop the pounds fast! However, most of the initial weight loss is water loss, rather than fat loss. With reduced consumption of carbohydrate in the diet, your body resorts to using its glycogen stores of glucose. Glycogen, which you store in your liver and muscles, can meet your glucose needs for about twelve to eighteen hours. With each gram of glycogen is stored 2.7 grams of water. An average body stores 300 grams of glycogen. Depletion of your glycogen stores will result in an almost overnight weight loss of three pounds. Combined with the strong diuretic effect caused by the ketones, you're looking at quick and dramatic weight loss. It is so seductive when you're desperate.

And the drama goes on. People on high-protein diets also lose weight because of the restriction of carbohydrate calories like those in fruits, vegetables, breads, pasta, cereals and beans. So many different foods are eliminated from their diet that their calorie intake is naturally reduced, even with all the calories present in meat, dairy and poultry. Anyone who has been on these wonder diets will agree that there is only so much steak you can eat before nausea sets in. So you get suckered in with promises of "unlimited meat, dairy and poultry" and the other "foods you love," but the truth is you can only eat so much. People on high protein diets are consuming up to 34% of their total calories from protein and a whopping 53% from fat, most of it saturated. But all of these diets restrict overall calories, so you lose weight. Of course, as people reach their ideal weight, some carbohydrate calories are added back into their diet as part of the maintenance plan, but should their weight begin to creep up (as it naturally will since they're adding calories), it's right back to the restricted diet. This way of losing weight seems hardly sustainable. Sure, there are the grim, determined few who have kept their weight off and have not had a piece of toast in years, but that is hardly living. The truth can't be denied. There is no magic potion, no magic pill; just calories in, versus calories out.

The other type of high-protein diet is the style that seriously limits the intake of food in general, like the famous (or infamous) Scarsdale Diet, the Zone Diet and the current Sonoma Diet. Well, duh! If your calorie intake is reduced to less than you expend, you will begin to lose weight. Conservative estimates of average caloric needs are around two thousand calories a day...and that's with only sedentary activity. Every day, on these types of plans, you're as much as one thousand calories short of your needs. Take away that many calories and what a surprise...you lose weight. The truth is that all calorie-restricted diets are next to impossible to sustain over a lifetime because it hurts to be hungry. Even though these high-protein diets claim there will be no hunger pangs because protein "stays with you longer," you begin to experience cravings (which are very real and very sucky) because your calorie intake and food options are so restricted. How happy is your life if you are miserable and hungry, thinking about food all the time?

Many credible experts point to the health, longevity and normalcy of weight of vegetarian cultures, while a diet centered around beef, pork, poultry, lamb, eggs, bacon, shrimp, lobster and dairy foods has been linked to just about every degenerative disease known to man, including obesity. Come on, people. It's time to admit that the reason these diets continue to thrive is that they give you permission to eat all the foods you know to be unhealthy...and that your intuition tells you are not right for you. These diets are like your own "Garden of Eden" of forbidden foods.

But look, if you think I'm nuts and still want to try a high-protein approach to dieting, then go with the South Beach Diet. At least this plan makes some nutritional sense, even though you will still be eating very large quantities of dead animals. I know the author is a cardiologist and I surely am not, but wow, all that saturated fat is keeping those guys working on your diseased hearts. So it's your choice.

SO WHAT DO WE DO?

All diets aren't nutty. Every single plan out there has something of value for the dieter. One extremely positive recommendation made by proponents of high-protein diets is their universal advice to avoid sugar, white flour, milk, ice cream, cakes, pies, soda and low-fat diet products that contain highly refined carbohydrates. Way too much sugar, baby. They also recommend a relatively high intake of healthy green and yellow vegetables, like asparagus, kale, collards and summer squash. Where they fail the dieter is by restricting your intake of essential complex carbohydrates, like brown rice, corn, beans and potatoes and by recommending butter, eggs, meats, and other very high-fat, high-cholesterol and/or high-protein foods. In the long run, these are not healthy choices. It really is that simple.

In and by itself, fat doesn't make you fat. Neither, in fact, do carbs, even the highly refined ones like sugar. And protein isn't quite the savior of the diet world that some would have you believe. What makes you fat is eating more calories than you burn—period.

THE NATURAL WAY

There is a natural way to achieve your ideal weight and to keep it under control without compromising your health. Just take a close look at cultures, societies and groups that maintain their weight without effort or diets. For instance, the traditional Japanese diet, particularly of the Okinawans, is abundant in rice and vegetables with only small amounts of animal protein. As a result, they have a very low incidence of heart disease, breast, colon and prostate cancer and the world's greatest longevity. Unfortunately, as Asian cultures adopt Western eating patterns of high-fat diets with lots of animal protein, they, too, are growing fat. But here's an interesting fact: When the Japanese government was given the news that 3% of their children were showing signs of obesity, they immediately took action to create healthier school lunches, control portions and discourage fast food and junk food intake. And that was when only 3% of their kids showed signs of trouble! We have close to two-thirds of our kids facing a lifetime of obesity and as a society, we do absolutely nothing but talk about it.

Another group, Seventh-day Adventists, many of whom are strict vegetarians and vegans, eat a diet that is mainly grains, legumes, fruits and vegetables. Research shows that they have a lower incidence of heart disease and colon cancer compared to the general population. A recent study of Seventh-day Adventists, and vegetarians in general, found that they lived longer and healthier and were not obese. For more than 130 years, this religious sect has practiced a vegetarian lifestyle because of their belief in the holistic nature of humanity. They believe that whatever is done with regard to eating and drinking should "glorify God" as it preserves the health of the body, mind and spirit. Regardless of your beliefs, it's sound thinking.

THE BEST DIET

So what comprises the best diet? I know I won't surprise you. Almost every expert of note agrees that, to stay healthy, we should eat a diet that is low in saturated fat and avoids *trans* fat, which means cutting out red meat, poultry, dairy food, sugar, hydrogenated fats and fast foods. A healthy diet is rich in vegetables and beans, whole cereal grains and pasta, whole wheat breads and crackers, fruit, nuts and seeds. The only real debate is how much oils or nut products or other foods that have unsaturated fats are necessary for good health. Certainly, some are necessary, not only for assimilation of fat-soluble nutrients, but to ensure that we get the right amounts of essential fatty acids. How much we need depends on our current condition of health, our activity level, our weight and our ancestry. Most experts agree that "good" fat is not only a healthy part of your diet, but essential to creating satisfaction. (See the section on fat in chapter 4.) And when you are satisfied by your food, you are far less likely to crave…or binge on foods that will ensure you stay fat and out of shape. Eating fat in a healthy way can help you find your way to the weight that is perfect for you.

The conclusion? Listen to that little voice inside you that always tells you the truth…your intuition. You'll discover your path to health and vitality is not rocket science and is paved with yummy food along the way.

The One Way to Lose

Let's be clear about one thing: There is only one way to lose weight. You must expend more calories than you take in. When your body has to draw on fat cells for fuel, you lose weight. Calories are simply units of energy. They provide us with the fuel we need to survive, but our bodies can only use so much energy. You know that taking in too many calories will make you fat because the body is storing that energy (in the form of fat)—sort of like your closet after you've gone on a shopping spree. If you keep shopping and don't recycle some of your old stuff, you've got a problem.

And you know that it's really easy to get fat and not so easy to lose it. There's a simple reason for that:

1 gram of protein contains 4 calories.
1 gram of carbohydrate contains 4 calories.
1 gram of fat contains 9 calories.

Carbohydrates are our primary source of fuel, stored in the body as glucose for easy access and fast use. And protein is stored as the body's last resort for fuel because its primary job is to *build* new tissue, not to provide fuel for activity. That's bad. If your body is relying on protein as fuel, it's easier for it to move into a toxic state, like ketosis, for survival. It will also be very difficult for you to gain and maintain strength, because the protein you eat is being used to fuel activity, not build muscle. Finally and most important, your body knows that it relies on muscle for survival so it will only use protein as a last choice for fuel because it needs that nutrient for other essentials to life, like movement and organ function, all of which rely on muscle function. Fat, on the other hand, is stored in the body as fatty acids to be used later. Your body has almost endless capacity to store any excess fat, and if you aren't using it (burning calories by exercise) then, guess what, you'll get fat. And, remember, fat has twice the calories of either carbohydrates or protein, so it's easy to gain weight.

A healthy diet of two thousand calories a day looks something like this: 45 to 65% of your daily calories need to come from carbohydrates for energy; 10 to 35% from protein to build new tissue and muscle; 20 to 35% from fat, with no more than 10% from saturated fat—and none of it from animal sources. That may seem like a lot of fat, but remember that fat is the vehicle that transports most of your nutrients to your cells, delivers flavor to your taste buds and keeps you satisfied so you will actually eat less. A well-balanced diet with this number of calories will maintain your body weight. To lose weight, you will need to drop that calorie count by two hundred to four hundred calories. If you reduce your intake by five hundred calories a day, things will move along a little more quickly. But you need to watch that you don't let your body get the message that you are starving it by eating too little. Your body will try to conserve energy if it thinks it faces starvation; metabolism will slow down and the scale will stay where it is. There's a fine line between reducing calories enough for steady weight loss and so much that your body won't release any fat, for fear of perishing.

EAT TO LOSE

You need to eat fewer calories, not necessarily less food. It's about the quality of the calories, not just quantity. But worry not; I will not condemn you to a life of celery sticks. Granted, celery is yummy and very light in calories (with lots of dietary fiber) but there are lots of choices you can make as alternatives to eating smaller amounts of calorically dense foods. You can stay within your calorie limits and not be hungry and cranky. Foods that are naturally lighter in calories allow you to eat until your heart is content, in more ways than one. But choosing "light" does not mean "lite," as in processed, packaged foods. I am not going to give you that easy way out. Why would you want to eat some junk snack that has been made "light" and then enriched with beta-carotene—just like carrots? Just eat the darn carrots! You get the crunch you want and the nutrients your body needs—and you did it as Mother Nature intended.

Let's say that you are allowing yourself sixteen hundred calories a day so you can lose some weight. Those calories must be spread out over all your meals and snacks for the day and keep you happy and satisfied. Not an easy task to begin with, but you're telling me that you love, love, love Sara Lee's Peanut Butter Thunder Cake. Well, just one 126-gram serving is 510 calories, with almost 50% of them from fat. If you want one of these (and I do not recommend it, truly…talk about a bad choice…), you will have used more than one-quarter of your calories for the day for one treat that goes down fast, but stays on your hips for months, maybe years. And if you think exercise is the answer, take note that you'll have to run about five miles at a five-minute mile pace to burn off that treat. Ouch!

Okay, so the tale of the peanut butter cake might be too obvious for you…of course you know you can't eat that stuff without consequences. We don't have to look at such an extravagant indulgence to get the picture. Take the common chicken breast, of which Americans eat zillions of pounds a year: a 3-ounce piece of roasted chicken breast (with the skin) is a mere 165 calories. Great news, right? Not so fast. Those calories are just for the chicken breast—no side dishes, no veggies, no salad, no bread, nada, niente—just chicken. It's not all that appealing. Instead, you could enjoy a luscious one-dish meal of stir-fried tofu with garlic, onions, carrots, and red peppers in a spicy peanut sauce over brown rice for just 142 calories, with no saturated fats, just deep, pat-your-tummy satisfaction. It looks as good as it tastes, which you couldn't say for the piece of beige chicken. You have to admit that rethinking your choices is making more sense with every page you read.

The Quality of Calories

If the calories we consume by choosing "low-fat" processed foods were doing the job, we'd all be thinner and fitter and healthier and not reading yet another book on how to be healthy, trim and fit. Do you really think that the nutrients in SnackWells and Diet Coke Plus are of the quality that your body can use to keep it healthy and strong?

The quality of calories in whole grains, beans, veggies, nuts, seeds, fruits and healthy oils are completely superior to those that you can get in a bucket of chicken parts, a steak or a hot dog. Your body needs fuel that it can use, stripped to its bare essentials in order to serve your needs properly. Whole, unprocessed calories, without the hindrance of chemical additives, pesticides, herbicides and saturated fat to muck up your body's functions, are those that will serve you best.

You must choose calories as close to their natural state as possible. And yes, meat can be natural, but with all the hormones, growth steroids, pesticides and other pollutants in it, do you really believe these are calories as Mother Nature intended?

TO ACHIEVE YOUR IDEAL WEIGHT, EAT YOUR VEGGIES

It's simple, really. If you want to lose weight for good, without deprivation and grim endurance of food; if you want to get and stay healthy, age gracefully and feel vital, you have to give up animal foods, junk and sugar. Period.

Now before you even start with the excuses, remember that I have heard them all. You don't teach healthy cooking for twenty years and not hear every bloody excuse that people can come up with as to why they can't eat well and give up foods that are making them sick and fat. So save your breath.

You look and feel best when you are properly nourished. That means a diet of vegetables, whole grains, beans, soy products, fruit and nuts. While it seems like a no-brainer, people always seem to be able to come up with one way or another to sabotage themselves. According to the American Dietetic Association, more than one-third of all adults routinely skip the healthy choice for some lame excuse. Let me guess. You're too busy to eat to sit down to a proper meal. You just crave foods that don't serve your health. (You like the taste of dinner in a bucket.) Your family gatherings are filled with fat-laden foods and you just can't be impolite. You don't like greens— and veggies are so much work to prepare. You won't get enough protein if you give up meat. (Did you even read chapter 4? Go back and review!) Well, Grasshopper, for every roadblock that you can create on your path to health, I have a nice and easy way to knock it down. Isn't that why you picked up this book in the first place?

Here are some of my favorite excuses from over the years—and some easy to live with solutions, so you can live a healthy, fit and slim life. No more complaining; no more whining. It's time to grow up…just a little…and eat well so you can enjoy a youthful vitality.

1. Veggies are so boring. They don't taste like anything. Rubbish, as my British friend says. Vegetables have lovely, nuanced flavors that may be hiding from you, but they are there. When you eat a diet rich in pro- cessed foods, sugar, soda, saturated fats, additives and preservatives, your taste buds become numbed to subtle flavors. So when you begin to eat veggies, some of their more delicate flavors may be lost on you. You think they're boring, but it's really you and your taste buds that need some fine- tuning. Give up all the high–saturated fat, high-salt, high-sugar foods for just twenty-one days and not only will you feel great and have lost weight, but you'll wonder what the farmers are putting in the soil. The veggies will taste that good to you.

There's more. Most people either overcook or undercook their vege- tables, leaving them bland and boring to the palate. When you are cook- ing vegetables, cook them just until they are tender, not until they can be pureed into baby food. On the other hand, make sure that you cook them enough to open the flavors and to make many of the nutrients available to your body for nourishment.

What do you do in the meantime? How do you get through the few weeks of "bland" flavors until your taste buds come alive? Cook your vegetables to perfect tenderness and then toss them with what chefs call a finishing sauce to coat them with a flavor that you like. This will help to make them more palatable to you until you grow to appreciate their many nuances. If you like sweet, whisk together a small amount of olive oil with balsamic vinegar, sea salt and pepper just enough to lightly coat the cooked vegetables. If spicy is your thing, toss them in a little hot sauce whisked together with olive oil, sea salt and pepper. And if you are the savory type, toss vegetables with a little herb mixture, such as Herbes de Provence or an Italian blend, or some finely minced fresh herbs, like chives and cilantro. There are also some lovely infused oils that you can buy, already flavored. Just be careful with them because they can deliver 120 calories in one tablespoon. That means twenty-four minutes of walking at a brisk pace! If you crave crunch, add a light sprinkle of pumpkin or sunflower seeds to your vegetables. You get the mouth feel you love and you add a dash of protein and healthy fat to your food.

Dressed up or plain, there's no excuse not to eat your veggies.

2. I don't have time for all the preparation and cooking that veggies need. Puh-leeze! If I had a nickel for every time I heard that one, I could retire. If you can find your way to the kitchen, you can cook vegetables. If you can tie your shoes, you'll be a master veg chef in no time! We're not splitting the atom here; we're steaming broccoli.

Seriously, cooking vegetables on a day-to-day basis is neither difficult nor time-consuming. Sure, if you are making a roasted vegetable dish for an evening meal, you will need to allow for an hour of oven time, but otherwise, vegetable dishes generally cook up in just minutes.

Take leafy greens...and I hope you do, every single day. If you have five minutes, you can have a delicious side dish on the table. Simply rinse the leaves, slice off the tips of the stems, steam or boil for two minutes, slice into bite-size pieces and you're done.

Want to make a stir-fry with lots of variety? You'll need fifteen minutes—twenty if you are really slow with a knife. Get your garlic and onions sliced and diced; heat a tiny bit of oil in a wok (or skillet); begin sautéing the garlic and onions. While they cook, slice and dice whatever other veggies you want into bite-size pieces and add them to the wok as they are prepped. From the cutting board to the wok, the prep and cook time is less than 30 minutes. If your health is not worth that to you, perhaps you need to rethink your priorities a bit, yes?

I could go on and on about how quick and easy it is to make vegetable dishes, but you'll find lots more ideas in the recipe section.

3. Fresh vegetables go bad before I eat them. Well, the first thing you have to do to combat this one is...eat veggies every single day. Most likely, the reason they spoil in the fridge is because...well...you didn't eat them!

Truthfully, most people buy way more than they need in a week's time, so make sure you only buy what you will use. This is where writing a week's worth of menu plans can really come in handy, especially if you are new to all this cooking and veg eating.

Ideally, you want to shop twice a week for the freshest vegetables and fruit you can get. For most of you, this may not be possible, so you need to look at your week and shop accordingly. Most vegetables are quite perishable and will only last about seven days, stored properly. Sure, you have winter squash, onions, carrots and other root veggies that can last a whole month or two, but for the most part, whatever vegetables you can't use in seven to ten days will most likely spoil. Figuring out how much to buy is easy, too. Kale or collards, very perishable leafy greens, will definitely not keep for more than a week, so if you know you will be using them daily, you can figure it this way: You'll be eating one to two leaves in a serving per person, so buy bunches with a good number of leaves. Gauge the amount that you buy on your appetite and how much you are cooking.

Next, store your abundance where you can see it. If you bury your delicate greens in the bottom of a crisper drawer or at the back of the fridge, chances are that you will forget to use them, because you don't have them in plain sight.

Storing produce properly is another essential tool for getting the most out of your purchases. Greens and delicate veggies, like salad ingredients, need to be stored in loosely closed plastic bags (the ones from the produce section, as they are designed to hold and release moisture as the veggies require to maintain freshness longer), while carrots and other hearty roots can be stored, unwrapped, in a crisper drawer. They are less likely to lose moisture, so wrapping them in plastic actually hastens spoilage. Onions, sweet potatoes, winter squash, bananas, avocadoes, tomatoes, lemons, limes, oranges, grapefruits, apples or pears do not even need refrigeration; just keep them in a bowl in a cool part of the kitchen. And keep the avocadoes and bananas away from all the other little fruits and veggies. They can outgas and hasten spoilage. Delicate fruits, like grapes, berries, apricots and peaches, however, need to be kept cold to stay fresh longer once they are ripe, so keep them in the fridge.

The "it goes bad so fast" excuse just got jettisoned. So let's head into the kitchen and get to work.

This Crazy Vegan Pantry

Now it's time to take stock—literally. With this book in hand, you'll be able to figure out what has to be on your shelves and in your fridge so that you can create a healthy vegan meal or snack quickly and easily.

First, you need to banish processed foods—which are not good at all. If the package label puts sugar or saturated fat at the top of the ingredient list, contains ingredients you can't pronounce or has an ingredient panel that reads like an epic novel, chances are it gets tossed or donated to a shelter (not that anyone needs to eat that food, but I hate waste). Second, you need to stock your kitchen with as much natural, fresh and organic food as your wallet (and availability) allows you to get.

These Crazy Vegan Staples

Let's keep this simple. As you cook and fall in love with your new life, you will naturally grow your list of staples and have all kinds of cool and crazy vegan stuff around to prepare great meals. For now, I just want to get you going with the basics. I consider my own pantry to be a food lover's paradise, with the shelves devoted to grains, beans, vinegars, miso and exotic spices and natural condiments, but the following list gives you the stripped-down version of what you would find if you opened my cupboard doors on any given day—and what I'd like to see in your kitchen. Chances are you already have a lot of these already, so now it's time to fill in the gaps, which you'll have because you'll be tossing some of the processed, packaged and refined stuff that's just taking up valuable space. (And don't worry if you aren't sure what some of these things are. I'll be talking about a lot of these things in the coming pages, and some have already been discussed in the previous chapters. So check the index of the book, visit your local health food store or go online to www.christinacooks.com for lots more information on ingredients.

- Extra-virgin olive oil
- Avocado oil
- Macadamia nut oil
- Dark sesame oil
- Red wine vinegar
- Brown rice vinegar
- Balsamic vinegar
- Organic soy sauce

- White unrefined sea salt
- Whole black peppercorns (in a pepper grinder)
- Crushed red pepper flakes
- Chili powder
- Curry powder
- Dried basil
- Dried oregano
- Dried thyme
- Saffron
- Ground cinnamon
- Whole or ground nutmeg
- Thai chili paste
- Dried cannellini beans
- Dried lentils (red, green and baby)
- Dried black beans
- Dried chickpeas
- Dried split peas
- Canned organic cannellini beans
- Canned organic black beans
- Canned organic chickpeas
- Canned organic diced tomatoes
- Marinated artichoke hearts
- Short-, medium- and long-grain brown rice
- Brown basmati rice
- Millet
- Quinoa
- Amaranth
- Barley
- Whole, steel-cut and rolled oats
- Kasha
- Farro
- Whole grain udon noodles
- Whole wheat pasta (in various cuts)
- Brown rice syrup
- Erythritol
- Pure vanilla extract
- Pure almond extract
- Whole wheat pastry flour
- Semolina flour
- Whole wheat flour
- Arrowroot or kuzu
- Baking powder
- Baking soda

THESE CRAZY VEGAN EXTRAS

I am pretty minimal when it comes to condiments and other stuff in my cooking besides what you see in the list above. Give me olive oil, sea salt, lemon and garlic any day of the week. But I love the flavors I can create with these ingredients, so they are nice to have around for those occasions when I want to give a dish a little something extra.

- Unsweetened organic ketchup
- Stone-ground and Dijon mustards

- Vegan "mayonnaise" (there are lots of brands; look for one without sugar)
- Barley, brown rice and sweet white miso
- Hot sauce (look for one without sugar)
- Oil-cured black olives
- Capers
- Marinated roasted red peppers
- Dried fruit (raisins, currants, apricots, prunes, etc.)

THIS CRAZY VEGAN FRIDGE

The pantry is important, to be sure. Yours has to be well-stocked so that you are not making your life insane trying to figure out meals. Most of us don't have time to shop every day, so keeping the pantry in good order is one less place for stress to live. The fridge is your focus for most meals since you will be working with fresh food that will give you vitality. Keeping the fridge well-stocked could mean shopping twice a week, but that's part of this crazy vegan life.

It's time to get past thinking of food shopping as a burden and look at it as you do any other shopping. Seeing it as an enjoyable task will remove the stress and help you stay focused on your goal. Take in all the colors; enjoy the fragrances of the fresh food. Bask in the life. Besides, you'll be spending so much of your time (and money) in the produce department that you will be infected by all the vitality just being there.

Several of the items that I've listed below do not need to be chilled (*) but can be kept beautifully displayed in bowls or baskets on your counter-top. You'll feel great just walking into your kitchen…

- Garlic (whole, not peeled or minced)*
- Yellow onions*
- Red onions*
- Scallions
- Leeks
- Fresh ginger*
- Parsley
- Basil (in season)
- Carrots
- Daikon
- Winter squash* (in season)
- Parsnips (in season)
- Turnips
- Rutabaga
- Yellow squash
- Zucchini
- Tomatoes (in season) *

- Cabbage (green and red)
- Chinese cabbage
- Cauliflower
- Broccoli
- Kale
- Collard greens
- Bok choy
- Watercress
- Arugula
- Escarole
- Broccoli rabe
- Lettuce (your choice)
- Cucumber
- Radishes
- Belgian endive
- Radicchio
- Frisée
- Fennel
- Bananas*
- Apples*
- Pears*
- Berries (in season)
- Melon (in season)
- Oranges*
- Tangerines*
- Lemons*
- Limes*

While these next items are not produce, they keep best in the fridge, so you will need to make room for:

- Whole grain bread
- Whole grain English muffins
- Sprouted whole grain breads

With your kitchen well-stocked, you will never find yourself standing like a deer in headlights facing the prospect of figuring out dinner. Just a little planning goes a long way toward making cooking, eating and living just a wee bit more fun.

Your Organic Kitchen

Your commitment to eating well begins with a change in thinking before you act. As you enjoy a meal, think about the food for a minute. Have you considered that the carrots you bought in the supermarket and are munching on as a snack may have traveled as many as fifteen hundred miles to get to you? That's a lot of fuel! Locally grown veggies and fruit, whether from a farm market or a supermarket (yes, some of them have locally produced food), helps to conserve energy, reduce pollution and support the existence of a local family farm...a win-win-win. And did I mention that locally produced food requires fewer preservatives like wax to keep it fresh?

Organic produce is grown with no pesticides, herbicides, fungicides or other chemicals and ensures the best quality you can buy. And with the pricing of organic produce falling right in line with most commercial options, the choice is clear. Or is it? If organic produce comes to your market from the other side of the country and is grown on a huge agri-giant of an organic farm, which is better? Organic or local? Now what do you do?

For me, the choice is not always clear cut. We are very blessed in my area of the world with farm markets, CSAs and local organic markets, all abundant with variety and choice. The bad news is that they are seasonal and when winter comes, I am back in the supermarket, in the organic produce section, buying the best quality I can get my hands on.

In my opinion, organic always trumps commercial. I want a better concentration of nutrients, like vitamin C, shown to be significantly higher in organic produce, and I want to know that the dollars I spend contribute to a sustainable way of growing food, protecting water from pollution, cutting down on erosion, conserving energy and saving the expense required to produce synthetic fertilizers and pesticides. But when I can find it, I go for locally produced organic fruits and veggies every time.

The bottom line? Do the best you can; seek out local and organic produce and enjoy.

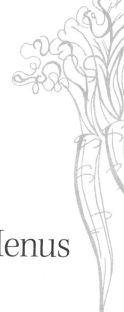

6

The Eating Plan: Menus and Recipes

No diet will remove all the fat from your body because the brain is entirely fat. Without a brain, you might look good, but all you could do is run for public office.

—GEORGE BERNARD SHAW

Your new life begins…now! It's time to get down to the business of achieving your ideal weight and great, vital health.

Any diet will produce results for you—at first. Most of them, sadly, fall apart in the long run. So why should you try this one? Why should you give up meat, fast food and all that "fun" stuff you are eating if diets fail in the long run? Because this is not a diet; this is a permanent lifestyle change. I am asking you to rethink your life. When you commit to that kind of change, your choices will change, too. The foods and lifestyle that are so comfy right now will simply no longer fit you. You wouldn't dream of wearing an old pair of bedroom slippers out on a hike. You old way of thinking and living just won't support the kind of transformation that's in store. You will come to love your new way of eating and how it makes you feel and look! There will be no more guilt, no more regret, no extra hours at the gym to work off excess and unnecessary calories. You will experience health and vitality you could not have imagined.

I have said it a million times in this book, but in case you skipped all the reading to get right down to the plan, I am saying it again. There is only one way to lose weight: You must take in fewer calories or burn off more. This simple law of nature forces your metabolism to make up the difference in what your body needs by tapping into your fat cells for fuel. You lose weight. It is the only way to succeed—*the only way.*

A healthy diet of 2,000 calories a day looks something like this: 45 to 65% of your daily calories need to come from carbohydrates for energy; 10 to 35% from protein to build new tissue and muscle; 20 to 35% from fat, with not 1% from trans or other unhealthy fats. The diet that I recommend in the following menu plans is one of weight loss, averaging 1,600 to 1,700 calories a day. You will need 2,000 calories a day (for women) and 2,400 calories a day (for men) to maintain your weight once you have reached your goal. By shaving off these calories, you will lose weight steadily and comfortably. But don't get carried away. Don't let your body get the message that you are starving it by eating too little. I have given you enough food and calories to keep you satisfied and still allow you to lose weight, so follow the plan. With the appropriate choices you can eat until you are well satisfied and cut your calorie intake substantially enough to lose the weight you want to lose. (See chapter 3, "Eat Well for Life," for details.)

Twenty-One Days to a New You

I have devised a twenty-one-day plan for you to re-create your health and wellness. In this plan, you will find easy to prepare, yummy recipes that will make your transition to a healthy, vegan style of eating much smoother. And yes, you can mix and match dishes to fit your tastes and your lifestyle. The key to crazy vegan living is to make this lifestyle fit you and who you want to be in the world. This plan is designed to serve as a guideline for you to change the way you relate to food.

A Simple Two-Phase Plan

This plan is divided into two phases: the first five days gets you started with a modified detox (don't worry, it sounds a lot scarier than it is); and the second reintroduces some foods that were eliminated, including more oil, pasta and breads.

An Overview of the Day-to-Day Menus

Breakfast

The breakfasts I recommend may be a little different for you—okay, a lot different. Most Americans are not used to savory breakfasts that feature veggies. Many people think nothing of having a vegetable omelet with a side of hash browns. I'm just asking you to let the veggies take center stage and skip the eggs. If you do it, at the end of even the first five days, you will wonder why you waited so long to get your act together for this meal.

Establish the habit of eating breakfast between 6:00 to 8:30 a.m. You must begin the process of creating habitual eating so that your metabolism will be stoked.

Lunch

Lunch is simple, but nutrient-dense and satisfying. Very low in fat, packed with complex carbs, protein and veggies to help you feel satisfied and strong, these simple meals give you all you need. While I have given you menu plans for this meal, you can substitute leftovers from the previous night's dinner to make your life easier on a workday. Just make sure that your calories stay in the same ballpark as the menu plan if you do that. When you want to substitute a dish, simply refer to it in the recipe section and see if its calories fit in with the rest of your day's eating. Keep in mind that a mere one hundred calories more than you need in a day will stall weight loss, so substitute accordingly.

Establish the habit of having lunch between noon and 1:30 p.m. Make your eating times as regular as possible to establish a rhythm for your body so that it "knows" that you are feeding it at regular intervals. I cannot stress this enough. You must eat at regular intervals for your metabolism to normalize.

Dinner

Your main meal is the time to refuel and relax after a long day. Your evening meal can be simple in structure, meaning that you don't need to make a dozen dishes, but has to include complex carbs, protein and veggies. Starting with a soup course is the best way to keep your appetite in check and your digestion clicking along happy and contented. (Too many of us fill up on bread at the beginning of a meal, especially when eating out—not a great move!)

Dinner can be eaten as early or late as your schedule demands, but remember to have your last meal of the day completed two to three hours before you go to bed. Be sensible here, too. If your schedule forces you to have dinner at 5:30 p.m., but you won't be retiring until close to midnight, save some calories for a snack at around 8:30 p.m., so you won't get cranky, wake ravenous or the worst scenario, go on a hunger-crazed eating binge during *The Daily Show.*

Snacks

Snacks are optional, but are nice to have on hand for those moments when the donuts in the coffee room are calling your name. They can also aid in keeping your metabolism stoked and burning. If you can keep from becoming ravenously hungry between meals, then you will be less likely to eat more than you need at the next one. Remember, though, these are snacks, not feasts. Keep them small yet satisfying—just a few bites to tide you over and keep hunger at bay.

You're going to want to take one of your two snacks midway between breakfast and lunchtime and an afternoon snack a couple of hours before dinner, but be flexible. If you are not hungry, don't snack; if you need something a little sooner than midway between meals, go for it. Just remember that your calories for the day are your calories for the day. In the following menus I have suggested some snack options but you can swap them in and out as you choose. Toward the end of the plan, I suggest that you have a Power Smoothie (page 257) as one of your snacks every other day, for added strength for your exercise. Just remember to keep tabs on your overall calorie counts for the day.

Home Remedies

Natural home remedies are a powerful aid in the battle of the bulge (and chronic disease, but that is another book). The remedies that I recommend for the next twenty-one days are simple, effective ways to help soothe the body from the inside out or kick-start your body's ability to break down and dispose of fat.

Carrot Daikon Drink (page 260), which resembles a hot soup, is dead-on effective in helping your body begin losing excess water weight and soft fat. You will be taking this remedy every other day for the first five days (in place of an afternoon snack) to get things moving. This is strong, so you only want to take it as recommended. Too much of this remedy can make you feel tired.

The other remedies, Kombu Tea (page 262) and Shiitake Tea (page 261) work deeper to help you to break down fat. Kombu is a sea plant with the unique characteristic of breaking down fat and protein in digestion, but it can also help to break down body fat like cellulite. Used in many spa treatments, kombu is a valuable tool in fat loss.

Shiitake Tea is made from delicate, dried shiitake mushrooms, which have the unique ability to break down stagnant, hardened fat in the body as well as lower cholesterol, cleanse plaque from veins and arteries and reduce blood pressure. Taken daily for the last eight days of the plan, this tea goes to work on the stubborn, hard fat that seems to take so much time and effort to lose.

Both Kombu and Shiitake Tea can be taken at any time of the day, but both must be taken hot.

And now you are ready to begin.

THE MENUS: PHASE I

These first five days are extremely important to kick-starting your weight loss and detoxification. Within this time period you will feel the beginnings of changes in your body. You'll feel clearer, fresher and lighter as toxins begin to leave your body. You will feel less achy and have more energy.

The simple home remedy in this phase, Carrot Daikon Drink, will accelerate your body's ability to get rid of excess, begin to cleanse your blood, and stimulate the process of creating a new you.

In these first five days, I have limited sweets. Let the whole grains and veggies work to stabilize your blood sugar and get rid of all the excess sugar floating around in your bloodstream. I have also minimized your use of oils, breads and pastas so that your digestion can strengthen and get used to the higher fiber content in your food. And last, I have used warm spices liberally—even curries—in order to stimulate circulation and get things moving, so to speak.

Use these five days to get your feet under you and lay some foundation for future health that doesn't include cravings.

Day 1

Think and Think Again A study presented to the American Heart Association showed that people adopting a vegetarian lifestyle lost more weight after eighteen months on a low-fat diet than those still eating meat, even on a low-fat diet—16.5 pounds versus 10.4 pounds. And their cholesterol normalized, too—without meds.

Breakfast

Breakfast Porridge, any variation
Daikon, Carrot and Winter Squash Stew
Steamed dark leafy greens, kale, collards or bok choy
        (2 cups raw, loosely packed)

Mid-Morning Snack *Choose one of the following:*

Tomato, Onion and Chile Salsa with rice cakes or celery sticks for dipping
1 Granny Smith apple with 2 tablespoons unsweetened peanut (or other nut or
        seed) butter

Lunch

Chickpea Soup with Smoked Paprika
Quinoa Tabouleh (without optional avocado)

Mid-Afternoon Snack/Home Remedy

Carrot Daikon Drink

Dinner

French Lentil and Vegetable Soup
Brown Rice and Vegetable Salad (without optional dressing)
Garlicky Collard Greens

⊚ *Crazy Vegan Tip of the Day* A daily body scrub (done in the shower or bath using hot water and a washcloth) is one of the most valuable tools for kick-starting weight loss; improving your circulation, sleep, and ability to handle stress; and enhancing concentration and overall vitality.

Day 2

Think and Think Again A food consultant in Michigan showed that people who regularly eat beans as a part of their daily diet weigh about seven pounds less than those who do not. The high-fiber content in beans helps the body digest fat more efficiently and makes people feel full more quickly so they eat less.

Breakfast
Miso Soup with Tofu
Amaranth and Corn
Steamed dark leafy greens (2 cups raw, loosely packed)

Mid-Morning Snack *Choose one of the following:*
1 Granny Smith apple with 2 tablespoons unsweetened peanut (or other nut or
　　seed) butter
1 Mini Pumpkin Cupcake

Lunch
Minestrone
Polenta with Spicy Sauteed Broccoli Rabe

Mid-Afternoon Snack *Choose one of the following:*
Cinnamon-Braised Apples
12 almonds

Dinner
Tofu and Red Pepper Stir-Fry over Quinoa
Mashed Sweet Potatoes with Orange
Cucumber-Radish Slaw with Mint Vinaigrette

◉ *Crazy Vegan Tip of the Day* Drinking enough water keeps you hydrated, prevents binge eating and is key to great skin. If you eat a largely plant-based diet, you take in lots of water with your veggies, so you may not need to drink the standard recommendation of eight glasses a day. While the right amount of water keeps you hydrated, too much leaves you looking washed-out—and there is a definite health risk to overhydrating.

Day 3

Think and Think Again Studies show that people consuming 800 mcg of folic acid daily for three years or more showed memory capacity of people five to seven years younger than those who did not. That's just ½ cup of cooked kale each day, my friends!

Breakfast
Breakfast Porridge, any variation
Daikon, Carrot and Winter Squash Stew
Steamed dark leafy greens, kale, collards or bok choy (2 cups raw, loosely
   packed)

Mid-Morning Snack *Choose one of the following:*
1 Granny Smith apple with 2 tablespoons unsweetened peanut (or other nut or
   seed) butter
2 cups air-popped popcorn, tossed with 2 teaspoons oil and ½ teaspoon sea salt

Lunch
Hot and Sour Tofu Soup
Herb-Scented Kasha Pilaf
Spiced Broccoli and Cauliflower

Mid-Afternoon Snack/Home Remedy
Carrot Daikon Drink

Dinner
Roasted Tomato and Chili Soup
Tortillas with Black Bean Sauce
Roasted Winter Squash with Basil
Asparagus Bundles

◉ *Crazy Vegan Tip of the Day* Cook extra food at dinner to use for lunch the next day—or as a head start on tomorrow's dinner. A pot of rice or other whole grain can create a couple of meals, from its first serving as a side dish, in a salad, in stir-fry or as the basis for morning porridge. Leftover vegetables are great to begin a soup, or puree them into a pâté for a snack.

Day 4

Think and Think Again A University of California, Berkeley, study revealed that diindolylmethane, a compound found in cruciferous vegetables like broccoli, kale, cabbage and cauliflower, boosts immune function while shutting down tumor growth. Only humble crucifers were shown to accomplish both these powerful jobs at one time. Broccoli, anyone?

Breakfast

Miso Soup with Tofu

Amaranth and Corn

Steamed dark leafy greens (2 cups raw, loosely packed)

Mid-Morning Snack *Choose one of the following:*

1 serving Edamame Hummus with celery and carrot sticks for dipping

2/3 cup Indian Rice Pudding

Lunch

Chickpea Puree and Fennel Salad

Garlic-Braised Broccoli

Mid-Afternoon Snack *Choose one of the following:*

1 Granny Smith apple with 2 tablespoons unsweetened peanut (or other nut or seed) butter

2 cups air-popped popcorn, tossed with 2 teaspoons oil and ½ teaspoon sea salt

Dinner

French Lentil and Vegetable Soup

Brown Rice and Vegetable Salad

Skinny Sweet Potato Fries

Garlicky Collard Greens

◉ *Crazy Vegan Tip of the Day* Water plays an important role in regulating your weight. Very often, what you perceive as hunger pangs could actually be thirst. Staying properly hydrated is just another insurance policy against bingeing. Most experts agree that drinking half your body weight in ounces is the best way to figure out what you need.

Day 5

Think and Think Again A study by Brandeis University shows that inter-esterified fats, the fats often used in place of trans fats, decrease your HDL (good) cholesterol and increase blood sugar by 30%, both of which boost your risk of heart disease.

Breakfast
Breakfast Porridge, any variation
Daikon, Carrot and Winter Squash Stew
Steamed dark leafy greens, kale, collards or bok choy (2 cups raw, loosely
    packed)

Mid-Morning Snack *Choose one of the following:*
Cinnamon-Braised Apples
2/3 cup Indian Rice Pudding

Lunch
French Lentil and Vegetable Soup
Farro Salad with Peas, Arugula and Tomatoes

Mid-Afternoon Snack/Home Remedy
Carrot Daikon Drink

Dinner
Gingered Squash Soup
Braised Tofu with Spring Greens and Pineapple-Curry Vinaigrette
Braised Baby Carrots and Tops

◉ *Crazy Vegan Tip of the Day* Staying hydrated need not burden our landfill even more than it is. Every day, more than 7 million plastic water bottles of varying sizes are thrown into the trash. Reuse your bottle for several days, refilling it at home. Buy water from the companies that make their bottles from recycled plastic—and recycle them when you are through with them.

The Menus: Phase II

By day five you should already be seeing some results. Your thinking is clearer; your body less achy. You've lost a couple of pounds. Now it's time to add some foods back into your plan to keep you interested and to make you more comfortable in this detox phase. As you change your diet (a big change for some), you may experience the discharge of toxins physically, like loose bowels for a day or so, a pimple or two, or even a headache. Keeping the detox phase to five days will keep you comfortable and still rid your body of toxins.

During these next sixteen days, as you get more familiar with a new style of cooking, you'll be able to be more flexible. I continue to include recommended dishes for each day and each meal, but if time is tight and you want to make lunch out of leftovers from yesterday's dinner, you'll figure out how to do that and still keep your calories in the same range with any substitutions.

I use oil, pasta and breads more abundantly in this phase, plus a sweet dessert or two. Breakfast does not change very much throughout the entire program. It is important that the habit of a soft grain and veggie breakfast become the foundation of your day. If you want to vary your grain or your veggies combos, have at it, but the structure of the meal should remain the same.

Day 6

Think and Think Again Australian researchers showed that meat eaters are more likely to suffer from squamous cell cancers than vegetarians. Apparently, the arachidonic acid in the saturated fat of meat contributes to the risk. The research also showed that fruit and vegetable eaters had a much lower risk due to vitamin E, selenium and carotenoids that occur in them.

Breakfast
Miso Soup with Tofu
Amaranth and Corn
Steamed dark leafy greens (2 cups raw, loosely packed)

Mid-Morning Snack *Choose one of the following:*
1 Mini Pumpkin Cupcake
1 Granny Smith apple with 2 tablespoons unsweetened peanut (or other nut or seed) butter

Lunch
Barbecued Tempeh Sandwich
Jicama Slaw with Mustard-Fennel Vinaigrette

Mid-Afternoon Snack *Choose one of the following:*
2 Taco Tarts
12 almonds

Dinner
Braised Carrot Soup
Basmati Rice with Curried Vegetables
Orange-Balsamic Glazed Tempeh over Greens
1 ounce dark chocolate

Home Remedy
1 cup Kombu Tea

◉ *Crazy Vegan Tip of the Day* The weekend is a good opportunity to make those dishes that require some extra effort or cooking time: a big pot of soup or beans or batches of cookies or muffins that can be frozen in individual portions to use during the week.

Day 7

Think and Think Again Statistics show that the average man in the United States has a 50% risk of a heart attack. He can reduce that risk by 45% by cutting his intake of meat by 50% and by 90% if he eliminates it all together.

Breakfast
Breakfast Porridge, any variation
Steamed broccoli and cauliflower (2 cups total)

Mid-Morning Snack *Choose one of the following:*
1 Granny Smith apple with 2 tablespoons unsweetened peanut (or other nut or seed) butter
Cinnamon-Braised Apples

Lunch
Fried Soba with Ginger and Scallion
Pan-Seared Tofu with Soy-Ginger Glaze

Mid-Afternoon Snack *Choose one of the following:*
2/3 cup Indian Rice Pudding
2 Taco Tarts

Dinner
Cannellini and Escarole Soup
Farro Salad with Peas, Arugula and Tomatoes
Asparagus Bundles

Home Remedy
1 cup Kombu Tea

⬤ *Crazy Vegan Tip of the Day* Eating out is a fact of life—but it doesn't have to sabotage your diet. On the day you will be eating out, be sure to have a great breakfast of whole grains and veggies. Eat a bit lighter than normal at lunch to conserve calories, but keep your mid-afternoon snack so that you are not ravenous by dinnertime. And last, the day you eat out is not the day to blow off your workout, as your metabolism will stay "revved" long after you have finished.

Day 8

Think and Think Again According to a 2005 study done at the University of Texas, El Paso, eating more than one-third of your calories at night results in weight gain. You tend to eat more because calories eaten at night are, curiously, less satisfying than those eaten during the day.

Breakfast
Miso Soup with Tofu
Quinoa Tabouleh (without avocado)
Steamed dark leafy greens (2 cups raw, loosely packed)

Mid-Morning Snack *Choose one of the following:*
Power Smoothie
Avocado and White Bean Dip with carrot sticks for dipping

Lunch
Curried Tofu Spring Rolls with Pineapple Sauce
Artichoke, Carrot and Zucchini Salad with Lime Vinaigrette

Mid-Afternoon Snack *Choose one of the following:*
Tomato, Onion and Serrano Salsa with 10–15 organic corn chips
1 ounce dark chocolate

Dinner
Curried Red Lentil Soup with Cilantro
Chili-Spiced Cornbread
Mustard-Scented Chickpea Salad
2/3 cup Indian Rice Pudding

Home Remedy
1 cup Kombu Tea

Crazy Vegan Tip of the Day Rather than slurping down a Fudgsicle or tearing open a bag of chips for your snack, choose something that makes you work for it a little. Try edamame (fresh soybeans in their pods), nuts in their shells, pomegranate, grapefruit or other fruit that requires peeling. You need to open each pod, crack each shell and take the time to peel. You'll eat more slowly and eat less as a result.

Day 9

Think and Think Again An Israeli study showed that the polyphenols in red wine reduce fat absorption in the body by as much as 30%. And you don't have to drink it; red-wine marinades work, too. Choose a vegan red wine and it's a win-win.

Breakfast

Breakfast Porridge, any variation

Daikon, Carrot and Winter Squash Stew

Mid-Morning Snack *Choose one of the following:*

2 Taco Tarts

1 Granny Smith apple with 2 tablespoons unsweetened peanut (or other nut or
   seed) butter

Lunch

Barbecued Tempeh Sandwich

Watercress and Avocado Salad with Basil Vinaigrette

Mid-Afternoon Snack *Choose one of the following:*

3 Chocolate-Coconut Macaroons

1 serving Edamame Hummus with celery and carrot sticks for dipping

Dinner

Winter Vegetable Bisque with Fresh Basil

Polenta with Spicy Sauteed Broccoli Rabe

Creamy Minted White Beans

Sauteed Brussels sprouts

Home Remedy

1 cup Kombu Tea

⬤ *Crazy Vegan Tip of the Day* I love to cook dried beans from scratch, letting them simmer for at least 1 hour, sometimes more, but I rely on canned organic beans for those nights when I need dinner in a hurry. Just rinse them well to remove any stale taste and excess salt, and serve them with lots of veggies for vitality.

Day 10

Think and Think Again A study from Wheeling Jesuit University in West Virginia showed that people who ate 3 ounces of dark chocolate before taking an academic test performed 20% better than those who did not. But it's not all good news. Three ounces of dark chocolate daily will pack on forty-seven pounds in a year. So, save up your chocolate binge for mid-terms, finals or that big presentation.

Breakfast
Miso Soup with Tofu
2 Citrus-Scented Seeded Muffins
Steamed broccoli and shredded green cabbage (2 cups total)

Mid-Morning Snack *Choose one of the following:*
1 Peanut Butter Cup
Cinnamon-Braised Apples

Lunch
Black Bean Burrito
Stir-Fried Bok Choy with Ginger and Garlic

Mid-Afternoon Snack *Choose one of the following:*
1 serving Hummus and Roasted Pepper Wrap
1 Granny Smith apple with 2 tablespoons unsweetened peanut (or other nut or
     seed) butter

Dinner
Curried Cauliflower and Yellow Split-Pea Soup
Quinoa and Sweet Potato Croquettes with Black Bean Salsa
Colorful Kale and Pepper Saute
1 Chocolate Peanut Butter Cookie or 1 ounce dark chocolate

Home Remedy
1 cup Kombu Tea

◉ *Crazy Vegan Tip of the Day* For some great advice on living a "greener" life, keeping up with the latest environmental news and finding some very cool vegan recipes, do yourself a favor and check out www.thedailygreen .com. Their daily e-newsletter is a great guide to all things green.

Day 11

Think and Think Again Complex carbohydrates like those found in brown rice protect your eyes from macular degeneration, according to the *American Journal of Clinical Nutrition*. Consumption of high-fiber, complex carb foods results in three times less risk of this leading cause of blindness in people over sixty-five. I hope you can see clearly that carbs are great for your health.

Breakfast
Breakfast Porridge, any variation
Steamed dark leafy greens (2 cups raw, loosely packed)

Mid-Morning Snack *Choose one of the following:*
1 slice Rustic Apple Tart
1 serving Hummus and Roasted Red Pepper Wrap

Lunch
Orecchiette with Green- and Black-Olive Pesto
Tomato Salad with Mint

Mid-Afternoon Snack *Choose one of the following:*
Power Smoothie
Sauteed Mushroom Crostini

Dinner
Miso Soup with Tofu
Basmati Rice with Curried Vegetables
Moroccan Lentil Stew
Steamed broccoli and cauliflower (2 cups total)

Home Remedy
1 cup Kombu Tea

⊙ *Crazy Vegan Tip of the Day* Eating Out, Redux: Order a salad with oil and vinegar or a simple veggie-based soup to start so that you fill up a bit before the main course. Enjoy a slice of bread, but hold off on eating the whole basket. Share a main course (most family-style restaurants serve portions that are much too large). And in spite of what your mother told you about starving children overseas, leave the leftovers.

Day 12

Think and Think Again The International Food Information Council states that America has a big, fat disconnect. Guidelines recommend consuming more poly- and monounsaturated fats, like those in vegetable oils, whole grains, avocadoes, nuts and seeds, but 42% of Americans surveyed said they were trying to cut down on these fats to be healthier, instead of eliminating the saturated fats they should be avoiding.

Breakfast

Miso Soup with Tofu
Breakfast Porridge, any variation
Daikon, Carrot and Winter Squash Stew

Mid-Morning Snack *Choose one of the following:*

1 Peanut Butter Cup
Cinnamon-Braised Apples

Lunch

Chickpea Soup with Roasted Paprika
Linguine al Verde

Mid-Afternoon Snack *Choose one of the following:*

Tomato, Onion and Chile Salsa with 10–15 organic corn chips for dipping
1 Granny Smith apple with 2 tablespoons unsweetened peanut (or other nut or
    seed) butter

Dinner

Herb-Scented Kasha Pilaf
Pan-Braised Tempeh with Tropical Salsa
Cauliflower with Cumin-Scented Oil
Steamed dark leafy greens (2 cups raw, loosely packed)

Home Remedy

1 cup Kombu Tea

◉ *Crazy Vegan Tip of the Day* If your time is tight in the morning, simply prepare your breakfast porridge and miso soup the night before. Then you just have to reheat them and steam your greens for 3 to 4 minutes.

Day 13

Think and Think Again High-fructose corn syrup, the insidious sweetener that is in 40% of all the food and beverages consumed by the average American, triggers overeating. It blocks the signal to your brain that you are full, so you lack appetite shut-off and can eat as much as 300 more calories than you need.

Breakfast
Breakfast Porridge, any variation
Boiled cauliflower, broccoli and carrot coins (2 cups total)

Mid-Morning Snack *Choose one of the following:*
1 serving Hummus and Roasted Red Pepper Wrap
Power Smoothie

Lunch
Brown Rice and Vegetable Salad
Baked Tofu with Moroccan Spices in Jicama-Ginger Slaw

Mid-Afternoon Snack *Choose one of the following:*
3 Chocolate-Coconut Macaroons
12 almonds

Dinner
Pinto Bean Chili with Fried Mushrooms
Chili-Spiced Cornbread
Cucumber-Radish Slaw with Mint Vinaigrette
2 Almond Cantucci

Home Remedy
1 cup Kombu Tea

◉ *Crazy Vegan Tip of the Day* When the weekend comes, you may have a little more time to make those dishes that you want to treat yourself to once a week, like Tomato Basil Pizza. These are great occasional foods, but shouldn't become the mainstay of your crazy vegan life. Remember that "occasional" means "now and then."

Day 14

Think and Think Again According to the International Food Information Council, 90% of Americans say that breakfast is a big part of healthy eating, but only 49% actually manage to eat it. And only 11% know how many calories they need each day to maintain a healthy weight.

Breakfast
Miso Soup with Tofu
1 slice whole grain toast with Spiced Onion Marmalade
Steamed dark leafy greens (2 cups raw, loosely packed)

Mid-Morning Snack *Choose one of the following:*
1 Mini Pumpkin Cupcake
1 Granny Smith apple with 2 tablespoons unsweetened peanut (or other nut or seed) butter

Lunch
Quinoa Tabouleh with Avocado
Stir-Fried Tofu with Soy-Simmered Shiitake and Wasabi

Mid-Afternoon Snack *Choose one of the following:*
1 serving Hummus and Roasted Pepper Wrap
2 Almond Bar Cookies

Dinner
Minestrone
Penne with Pan-Roasted Tomato-and-Chili Sauce
Bitter Greens Salad with Walnut-Shallot Vinaigrette

Home Remedy
1 cup hot Shiitake Tea

Crazy Vegan Tip of the Day Certified organic foods do not contain any genetically modified organisms (GMOs) and are produced without pesticides, herbicides, fungicides and other toxins. You may also see "GMO-Free" on labels of products that are not organic, but there are no regulations for the use of this label. Find out everything you need to know about GMOs and labeling by going to the True Food Shopping List at www.truefoodnow.org.

Day 15

Think and Think Again A 2007 Cornell University study (published in *International Journal of Impotence Research*) revealed that regular consumption of pure pomegranate juice may be a powerful erection enhancer. The potent antioxidant concentration increases blood flow to the male genital area by removing plaque from the arteries. Potent indeed.

Breakfast
Amaranth and Corn
Daikon, Carrot and Winter Squash Stew

Mid-Morning Snack *Choose one of the following:*
Power Smoothie
1 serving Hummus and Roasted Pepper Wrap

Lunch
Fried Tempeh over Cold Sesame Noodles
Prune, Orange, Red Onion and Fennel Salad

Mid-Afternoon Snack *Choose one of the following:*
1 ounce dark chocolate
Tomato, Onion and Chile Salsa with 10–15 organic corn chips for dipping

Dinner
Hot and Sour Tofu Soup
Basmati Rice with Curried Vegetables
Fresh Fava Bean, Onion and Fennel Saute
Frisée, Escarole and Dulse Salad
1 slice Steamed Pear Pudding

Home Remedy
1 cup hot Shiitake Tea

◉ *Crazy Vegan Tip of the Day* As the meaning of the word *organic* is diluted by big business, it's important that you understand terms like *sustainable*, as farmers and small producers struggle to retain a foothold on their business. Sustainable refers to ways of growing, raising and producing food that has minimal impact on the environment, with the farm seen as an extension of the local community.

Day 16

Think and Think Again A 12-ounce regular soda has 10 to 13 teaspoons of sugar and more than 160 empty calories. That yummy margarita has more than 200 calories in 4 ounces, your daiquiri has more than 224 in 4 ounces. And that Dunkin' Donuts Mocha Hot Almond Latte you think you deserve? It comes with a whopping 290 calories for a 10-ounce serving. Time to drink smarter.

Breakfast
Miso Soup with Tofu
Breakfast Porridge, any variation
Steamed dark leafy greens (2 cups raw, loosely packed)

Mid-Morning Snack *Choose one of the following:*
1 Peanut Butter Cup
Cinnamon-Braised Apples

Lunch
Nut-Crusted Tofu with Szechuan-Style Vegetables
Braised Kale Crostini

Mid-Afternoon Snack *Choose one of the following:*
Guacamole with Roasted Tomato and Garlic with 10–15 organic corn chips for
    dipping
1 Granny Smith apple with 2 tablespoons unsweetened peanut (or other nut or
    seed) butter

Dinner
French Lentil and Vegetable Soup
Tomato Basil Pizza
Braised Endive and Pear Slices with Lemon

Home Remedy
1 cup hot Shiitake Tea

⊙ *Crazy Vegan Tip of the Day* You'll be using a lot of little snack bags to freeze cookies, muffins and other treats in small servings, as well as to transport snacks to work. Don't just dump them into the landfill. Take them home; wash them with warm, soapy water; rinse well and hang them on your kitchen faucet to dry. You'll save money and the environment.

Day 17

Think and Think Again The *Journal of Clinical Endocrinology and Metabolism* says that a four-point increase in a man's body mass index (BMI) will acceler-ate the decline of testosterone production by ten years. That's thirty pounds of gut on a 5'10" man. Yikes; no wonder 40% of all women are more turned on by thoughts of chocolate than kissing, and no wonder Viagra and Cialis are doing so well in our world.

Breakfast
2 Citrus-Scented Seeded Muffins
Daikon, Carrot and Winter Squash Stew

Mid-Morning Snack *Choose one of the following:*
Power Smoothie
2 Taco Tarts

Lunch
Tofu, Red Pepper and Asparagus Stir-Fry over Quinoa

Mid-Afternoon Snack *Choose one of the following:*
12 almonds
1 serving Edamame Hummus with 1/2 whole wheat pita bread for dipping

Dinner
Cannellini and Escarole Soup
Polenta with Spicy Sauteed Broccoli Rabe
Cauliflower in Spiced Tomato Sauce
2 Pignoli Cookies

Home Remedy
1 cup hot Shiitake Tea

◉ *Crazy Vegan Tip of the Day* Join a Community Supported Agri-culture. A CSA allows members to own a "share" of a farm as a way for them to develop a relationship with the small family farm that grows their food. With weekly pickups, you are guaranteed the freshest and most alive local, often organic, produce you can get. Your financial commitment ensures that you get your share of the crop and helps the small family farm stay in business. It's a win-win. Go to www.localharvest.org to find a CSA near you.

Day 18

Think and Think Again One ten-piece McDonald's Chicken Select Breast Strips with Barbecue Sauce has 1,030 calories. You'd have to run the length of a football field 109 times to burn those babies off. One Baskin-Robbins Banana Split also has 1,030 calories. You'll need to swim for 125 minutes in rough surf to reverse the damage done to your waistline. And that Ruby Tuesday's Smokehouse Burger and Fries? It weighs in at 1,751 calories! But you can run just 12.4 miles and you'll never know you had it.

Breakfast
Miso Soup with Tofu
Breakfast Porridge, any variation
Steamed dark leafy greens (2 cups raw, loosely packed)

Mid-Morning Snack *Choose one of the following:*
3 Chocolate-Coconut Macaroons
1 Granny Smith apple with 2 tablespoons unsweetened peanut (or other nut or
   seed) butter

Lunch
Barbecued Tempeh Sandwich
Skinny Sweet Potato Fries
Boiled broccoli (1 cup florets)

Mid-Afternoon Snack *Choose one of the following:*
1 serving Hummus and Roasted Pepper Wrap
1 Mini Pumpkin Cupcake

Dinner
Gingered Squash Soup
Farro Salad with Peas, Arugula and Tomatoes
White Beans with Sage and Oil
Garlicky Collard Greens

Home Remedy
1 cup hot Shiitake Tea

◉ *Crazy Vegan Tip of the Day* Wrap your sandwich ingredients in a leaf of Romaine or Bibb lettuce instead of bread and save an average of two hundred calories for that meal.

Day 19

Think and Think Again A 2004 Finnish study (published in the *Journal of the American Medical Association*) showed that people who drank just 6 ounces of soda a day raised their risk of diabetes by 67%. That's half a can, baby. This stuff is so lethal for your health you don't even need to finish a serving to do all the damage!

Breakfast
Buckwheat Pancakes with Red Chile Syrup or Fruit Salsa

Mid-Morning Snack *Choose one of the following:*
Power Smoothie
1 serving Hummus and Roasted Pepper Wrap

Lunch
Brown Rice and Vegetable Salad
Braised Tofu with Spring Greens and Pineapple Vinaigrette

Mid-Afternoon Snack *Choose one of the following:*
1 serving Maple Popcorn (or plain air-popped popcorn)
12 almonds

Dinner
Braised Carrot Soup
Quinoa and Sweet Potato Croquettes with Black Bean Salsa
Artichoke Stew with Peas
1 serving Cinnamon-Pear Crisp

Home Remedy
1 cup hot Shiitake Tea

⦿ *Crazy Vegan Tip of the Day* A combination of the herbs calendula and chamomile can relieve the inflammation that causes skin breakouts and pimples. Mix 1 tablespoon of each dried herb in 1 cup boiling water and steep until room temperature. Do not cool in the refrigerator, as it will weaken the brew. Using a fresh cotton ball, dab this gentle herbal potion on the blemishes. Don't rinse. This brew will keep, refrigerated, for five days.

Day 20

Think and Think Again Common ingredients can extend and improve the quality of your life. Extra-virgin olive oil is a rich source of anti-aging antioxidants; dark chocolate contains flavenols, shown to reduce the risk of heart disease. Studies show that people who eat nuts on a daily basis live 2½ years longer than those who do not. Simple, sweet blueberries are such a rich source of antioxidants that they can extend your life by 3 years. A glass of red wine has reservatrol, a powerful anti-aging compound.

Breakfast
Miso Soup with Tofu
Millet with Cinnamon Onions
Daikon, Carrot and Winter Squash Stew

Mid-Morning Snack *Choose one of the following:*
1 Mini Pumpkin Cupcake
1 Granny Smith apple with 2 tablespoons unsweetened peanut (or other nut or seed) butter

Lunch
Black Bean Burrito
Bitter Greens Salad with Walnut-Shallot Vinaigrette

Mid-Afternoon Snack *Choose one of the following:*
Tomato, Onion and Chile Salsa with 10–15 organic corn chips for dipping
2 Almond Bar Cookies

Dinner
Roasted Tomato and Chile Soup
Orecchiette with Green- and Black-Olive Pesto
Lentils with Greens

Home Remedy
1 cup hot Shiitake Tea

◉ *Crazy Vegan Tip of the Day* The weekend usually gives you a little more time to spend at the stove, but some advance planning always helps. Millet takes only 30 minutes to cook, but the lovely cinnamon-scented onions take 1 hour. Simply prep and roast the onions the night before while you make dinner, and just stir them into your millet for a delightful breakfast cereal.

Day 21

Think and Think Again Your La-Z-Boy recliner may make you look more like one than you think. Studies at the University of Missouri conducted in 2007 show that sitting shuts down your fat burners. The study concluded that parking your butt turns off the enzyme that prevents fat storage. So, take a break from your desk work or that *Law and Order* marathon. Just a few minutes of activity every hour will keep your metabolism burning.

Breakfast
Amaranth and Corn
Boiled broccoli and cauliflower (2 cups total)

Mid-Morning Snack *Choose one of the following:*
Power Smoothie
1 Granny Smith apple with 2 tablespoons unsweetened peanut (or other nut or seed) butter

Lunch
Pinto Bean Chili with Fried Mushrooms
Chili-Spiced Cornbread
Colorful Kale and Pepper Saute

Mid-Afternoon Snack *Choose one of the following:*
1 serving Hummus and Roasted Pepper Wrap
12 almonds

Dinner
Minestrone
Artichokes Stuffed with Gremolata
Tangy Pear and Blueberry Salad
1 Peanut Butter Cup or 1 ounce dark chocolate

Home Remedy
1 cup hot Shiitake Tea

◉ *Crazy Vegan Tip of the Day* There is nothing like a Sunday morning run followed by a serving of Buckwheat Pancakes or Better French Toast with Fruit Salsa. I love my whole grain and veggie breakfasts during the week, but I love these treats on the weekend, too. They make for a nice balance.

THE RECIPES

About the Nutritional Analysis

All recipes were analyzed using the Food Processor, Version 8.1, software program. Any ingredients that are to taste, such as salt and pepper, or are optional, are not included in the analysis. When there is a choice of ingredients in a recipe, the first ingredient is used for the analysis. If an ingredient was not listed on the database, then a similar product with similar nutritional content was used for the analysis. When a recipe yield is a range, such as 2 or 3 servings or 4 to 6 servings, the first number is used. If you divide the recipe into the larger number of servings, the calorie count and other values will be slightly less.

SOUP OF THE DAY

Served at the top (as we say in our house) as an appetizer, soup sets the tone for the rest of the meal. Prepared according to the principles of balance, the taste, texture, fragrance and ingredients should all complement the other dishes being served.

If a meal is simple and light, then your soup should be richer and more satisfying. If the main meal is decidedly hearty fare, then your soup should be light and simple to balance out the richness of the courses to follow.

Soup plays a key role in a healthy diet year round. In cool weather, hearty soups and stews, thick with grains, beans and chunks of veggies, make us feel warm, cozy and satisfied. In warmer weather, lighter soups with leafy greens, shiitake mushrooms and delicately sliced vegetables will make us feel cool, comfortable and relaxed. A bowl of soup on even the hottest day will refresh you, just as it warms you to your toes in the depths of winter.

In my kitchen, soup is made fresh every day, except for bean-based soups, which improve with a day's aging. You can also make a variety of soups when you have an open day and freeze them in serving-size portions. You'll have a variety of "fresh" soups, with more time to spend on the rest of the meal—or with the family.

When you are making soups, you will always want to begin with a good base. I am not a fan of using traditional stock but you can decide and use them as you like. I almost always begin with sautéing garlic, herbs, onions, celery and carrot (or some variation of those ingredients) in a little olive oil. Called *soffritto* in Italian cooking or *mirepoix* in French cuisine, these ingredients create the base on which you build your soup. You will note in the recipes that I add an ingredient and a pinch of salt and cook each item for a minute or so before adding the next. This technique helps you create depth of flavor while allowing each ingredient to maintain its own character.

After you've tried some of these soups, you'll never think about picking up a can opener again.

Hot and Sour Tofu Soup

MAKES 4 TO 5 SERVINGS

4 dried shiitake mushrooms

4–6 dried maitake mushrooms

5½ cups spring or filtered water

3–4 tablespoons soy sauce

5 tablespoons brown rice vinegar

¼ cup arrowroot

4 ounces extra-firm tofu, sliced into ¼-inch strips

½ teaspoon hot chili oil

1 teaspoon avocado oil

½ yellow onion, cut into thin half-moon slices

2 stalks celery, thinly sliced on the diagonal

Generous pinch crushed red pepper flakes

½ teaspoon ground black pepper

Generous pinch ground white pepper

2–3 scallions, thinly sliced on the diagonal

Place shiitake and maitake mushrooms in a bowl and cover with 2 cups of the water. Soak until soft, about 30 minutes. Slice the mushrooms thinly and reserve the soaking water.

Whisk together 3 tablespoons soy sauce, brown rice vinegar and arrowroot. Lay tofu strips in a shallow dish and spoon soy sauce mixture over top, covering completely. Allow to marinate for 10 minutes. Drain and reserve marinade.

Heat oils in a soup pot over medium heat. Add onion, celery and red pepper flakes and sauté for 2 minutes. Add remaining 3½ cups water, ½ cup of the reserved mushroom soaking water (leaving any sand in the bottom of the bowl), mushrooms and tofu and bring to a boil. Cover and reduce heat to low. Cook until mushrooms are tender, 25 to 30 minutes. Season with black and white peppers; stir in 3 to 4 tablespoons of the reserved tofu marinade. Simmer for 5 minutes. Serve garnished with scallions.

PER SERVING: Calories 93; Protein 4.4g; Total Fat 2.6g; Saturated Fat .34g; Cholesterol 0mg; Carbohydrate 13.7g; Dietary Fiber 1.1g; Sodium 707mg

Braised Carrot Soup
MAKES 4 TO 6 SERVINGS

4 teaspoons extra-virgin olive oil

1 tablespoon balsamic vinegar

1½ teaspoons sea salt, plus additional to taste

6–8 carrots, small-chunk cut

½ yellow onion, diced

2 Yukon gold potatoes, peeled, diced

Scant pinch ground nutmeg

4 cups spring or filtered water

2 sprigs fresh mint, leaves removed and finely shredded

Place 2 teaspoons of the oil, vinegar and ½ teaspoon salt in a large, flat-bottomed skillet over medium heat. Arrange carrots in oil mixture, avoiding overlap as much as possible. Cover and listen closely for a strong sizzle. When you hear the sizzle, reduce heat to low and cook until carrots are tender and the liquid has become a thick syrup, 15 to 20 minutes (depending on the size of the carrot pieces).

In a large saucepan, place remaining 2 teaspoons oil and onion over medium heat. When the onion sizzles, add a pinch of salt and sauté for 1 to 2 minutes. Add potatoes, nutmeg, braised carrots and water. Bring to a boil, cover and reduce heat to low. Cook until potatoes are tender, about 20 minutes. Season with about 1 teaspoon salt and simmer for 5 minutes more.

Transfer soup by ladles to a food processor and puree until smooth. Return to pot and warm through. Serve garnished with mint.

PER SERVING: Calories 134; Protein 2.2g; Total Fat 4.9g; Saturated Fat .68g; Cholesterol 0mg; Carbohydrate 21.2g; Dietary Fiber 4.3g; Sodium 900mg

Roasted Tomato and Chile Soup

MAKES 7 SERVINGS

2 pounds plum tomatoes, cut into large dice

6 cloves fresh garlic, peeled, left whole

½ red onion, largely diced

1 small serrano chile, seeded, diced

2 teaspoons extra-virgin olive oil

1 tablespoon balsamic vinegar

½ teaspoon sea salt, plus additional to taste

Generous pinch cracked black pepper

6–8 fresh basil leaves

2 cups spring or filtered water

Basil sprigs, for garnish

Preheat oven to 375 degrees.

Place tomatoes, garlic, onion and chile in a mixing bowl. Stir in olive oil, balsamic vinegar, salt and pepper until coated. Spread the vegetables on a shallow baking sheet, avoiding overlap. Roast, uncovered, about 45 minutes, until the vegetables are tender.

Transfer roasted vegetables to a food processor and puree until smooth. Transfer pureed tomato mixture to a soup pot and add water. Bring to a boil, and season with salt. Stir in basil leaves, reduce heat to low and cook for 5 to 7 minutes.

Serve garnished with basil sprigs.

PER SERVING: Calories 47; Protein 1.4g; Total Fat 1.7g; Saturated Fat .25g; Cholesterol 0mg; Carbohydrate 7.9g; Dietary Fiber 1.6g; Sodium 177mg

Gingered Squash Soup

MAKES 4 SERVINGS

2 teaspoons avocado oil

1 yellow onion, diced

1 clove fresh garlic, minced

2 teaspoons fresh grated ginger

Sea salt

2 cups diced butternut squash

2½ cups spring or filtered water

½ cup fresh orange juice

2 teaspoons grated fresh orange zest

Scant pinch nutmeg

Cracked black pepper

3 sprigs flat-leaf parsley, finely diced

Place oil in a medium saucepan over medium heat. Add onion, garlic, ginger and a pinch of salt and sauté until onion is translucent, about 3 minutes. Add squash, water, orange juice, zest and nutmeg and bring to a boil. Cover, reduce heat to low and cook until squash is quite soft, about 20 minutes. Season with about 1 teaspoon salt and pepper and simmer 3 minutes more.

Ladle soup into a food processor and process until smooth. (You may also use a food mill or chinois and puree by hand.) Return soup to pan and simmer until ready to serve. Serve garnished with parsley.

Note: To save about 15 calories, use only water and eliminate the orange juice. The zest will give you plenty of orange flavor.

PER SERVING: Calories 79; Protein 1.3g; Total Fat 2.5g; Saturated Fat .3g; Cholesterol 0mg; Carbohydrate 14.4g; Dietary Fiber 3g; Sodium 614mg

Winter Vegetable Bisque with Fresh Basil

MAKES 4 TO 5 SERVINGS

1 teaspoon avocado oil

½ red onion, diced

Sea salt

1 carrot, diced

1 stalk celery, diced

1 parsnip, diced

1 cup diced butternut squash

1 cup diced green cabbage

1 small sweet potato, diced

4 cups spring or filtered water

1 bay leaf

2 teaspoons sweet white miso

Scant pinch fresh nutmeg

2 stalks fresh basil, leaves removed and shredded

Heat oil in a soup pot over medium heat. Add onion and a pinch of salt and sauté until translucent, about 3 minutes. Stir in carrot and a pinch of salt and sauté for 1 minute. Stir in celery and a pinch of salt and sauté for 1 minute. Stir in parsnip and a pinch of salt and sauté for 1 minute. Stir in butternut squash and a pinch of salt and sauté for 1 minute. Stir in cabbage and a pinch of salt and sauté for 1 minute. Stir in sweet potato and a pinch of salt and sauté for 1 minute. Add water and bay leaf and bring to a boil. Cover and reduce heat to low. Cook until vegetables are tender, about 30 minutes. Remove bay leaf and discard.

Ladle soup into a food processor and puree until smooth. (You may also use a food mill or chinois.) Return to pan. Remove a small amount of soup and stir in miso until dissolved. Stir miso mixture and nutmeg into soup and simmer for 3 to 4 minutes more. Serve garnished with basil.

PER SERVING: Calories 87; Protein 1.8g; Total Fat 1.5g; Saturated Fat .18g; Cholesterol 0mg; Carbohydrate 18g; Dietary Fiber 4g; Sodium 390mg

French Lentil and Vegetable Soup

MAKES 4 TO 5 SERVINGS

1 teaspoon extra-virgin olive oil

2 cloves fresh garlic, finely minced

½ red onion, diced

Sea salt

2 stalks celery, diced

1 medium carrot, diced

1 cup LePuy lentils, rinsed very well

1 cup canned diced tomatoes

4 cups spring or filtered water

1 bay leaf

2 stalks flat-leaf parsley, coarsely minced, for garnish

Place oil, garlic and onion in a medium pot over medium heat. When the onion begins to sizzle, add a pinch of salt and sauté until translucent, about 3 minutes. Stir in celery and a pinch of salt and sauté for 1 minute. Stir in carrot and a pinch of salt and sauté for 1 minute. Add lentils, tomatoes, water and bay leaf and bring to a boil. Cover and reduce heat to low. Cook until lentils are soft, about 45 minutes. Season with about 1 teaspoon salt and simmer 5 to 7 minutes more. Remove and discard bay leaf. Serve garnished with parsley.

PER SERVING: Calories 202; Protein 14.5g; Total Fat 1.7g; Saturated Fat .25g; Cholesterol 0mg; Carbohydrate 34.3g; Dietary Fiber 16.7g; Sodium 999mg

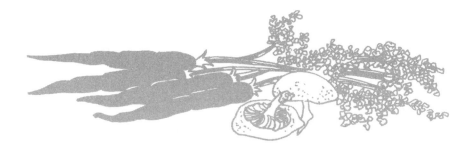

Cannellini and Escarole Soup

MAKES 4 TO 5 SERVINGS

2 teaspoons extra-virgin olive oil

2 cloves fresh garlic, finely minced

½ yellow onion, diced

Sea salt

Generous pinch crushed red pepper flakes

1 cup thinly sliced cremini mushrooms

1 cup cannellini beans, rinsed well, soaked for 1 hour in hot water

4 cups spring or filtered water

1 bay leaf

2 teaspoons sweet white miso

5–6 leaves escarole, rinsed very well, hand-shredded into bite-size pieces

Place oil, garlic and onion in a medium pot over medium heat. When the onion begins to sizzle, add a pinch of salt and red pepper flakes and sauté until translucent, about 3 minutes. Stir in mushrooms and a pinch of salt and sauté until just wilted, about 3 minutes.

Drain beans and discard soaking water. Add beans, water and bay leaf to the pot and bring to a boil. Cover and reduce heat to low. Cook until beans are quite soft, about 1 hour. Remove and discard bay leaf. Remove a small amount of broth and stir in miso until dissolved. Stir miso mixture and escarole into soup and simmer for 3 to 4 minutes more.

Note: You can shorten your cooking time on this soup to 30 minutes by using canned organic cannellini beans. Just rinse them well before use to remove any stale flavor and excess salt from the water in the can.

PER SERVING: Calories 191; Protein 10.6g; Total Fat 2.9g; Saturated Fat .5g; Cholesterol 0mg; Carbohydrate 31.6g; Dietary Fiber 9.9g; Sodium 160mg

Chickpea Soup with Smoked Paprika

MAKES 4 TO 5 SERVINGS

1 teaspoon extra-virgin olive oil

2 cloves fresh garlic, finely minced

½ red onion, diced

Sea salt

Generous pinch smoked paprika (see Note, page 148)

2 stalks celery, diced

1 medium carrot, diced

1 small parsnip, diced

½ cup diced green cabbage

1 cup chickpeas, rinsed well, soaked for 1 hour in hot water

4 cups spring or filtered water

1 bay leaf

2–3 scallions, thinly sliced, for garnish

Place oil, garlic and onion in a medium pot over medium heat. When the onion begins to sizzle, add a pinch of salt and sauté until translucent, about 3 minutes. Stir in smoked paprika to coat the onion. Stir in celery and a pinch of salt and sauté for 1 minute. Stir in carrot and a pinch of salt and sauté for 1 minute. Stir in parsnip and a pinch of salt and sauté for 1 minute. Stir in cabbage and a pinch of salt and sauté for 1 minute.

Drain chickpeas and discard soaking water. Add chickpeas, water and bay leaf and bring to a boil. Cover and reduce the heat to low. Cook until chickpeas are tender, about 1 hour, but it could take as long as 90 minutes. (Chickpeas can have a mind of their own.) Season with about 1 teaspoon salt and simmer 5 to 7 minutes more. Remove and discard bay leaf. Serve soup garnished with scallions.

Note: You can cut your cooking time to 30 minutes if you use canned organic chickpeas instead of cooking them from scratch. Just rinse the beans well to avoid the stale taste and excess salt that can come from the water in the can.

Note: Smoked paprika can be purchased anywhere that spices are sold. If you can't find it, go with regular sweet paprika.

PER SERVING: Calories 214; Protein 10.9; Total Fat 3.3g; Saturated Fat .19g; Cholesterol 0mg; Carbohydrate 36.8g; Dietary Fiber 8.2g; Sodium 757mg

Curried Cauliflower and Yellow Split-Pea Soup
MAKES 4 TO 5 SERVINGS

2 teaspoons avocado oil
½ yellow onion, diced
3 cloves fresh garlic, crushed
Sea salt
1 teaspoon curry powder
2 cups diced cauliflower
1 cup yellow split peas, rinsed well
4 cups spring or filtered water
1 bay leaf
2 sprigs cilantro, finely minced, for garnish

Heat oil in a medium pot over medium heat. Add onion, garlic and a pinch of salt and sauté until onion is translucent, about 3 minutes. Stir in curry powder until onion is coated and bright yellow. Stir in cauliflower and a pinch of salt and sauté for 1 minute. Add split peas, water and bay leaf and bring to a boil. Cover and reduce heat to low. Cook until the split peas are creamy and soft, 45 minutes to 1 hour. Season with about 1 teaspoon salt and simmer for 5 to 7 minutes more. Remove and discard bay leaf. Serve garnished with cilantro.

PER SERVING: Calories 210; Protein 13.3g; Total Fat 3.2g; Saturated Fat .4g; Cholesterol 0mg; Carbohydrate 35.3g; Dietary Fiber 14g; Sodium 694mg

Minestrone

MAKES 5 TO 6 SERVINGS

1 teaspoon extra-virgin olive oil
2 cloves fresh garlic, finely
    minced
½ yellow onion, diced
Sea salt
Cracked black pepper
½ small leek, diced, rinsed
    very well
1 stalk celery, diced
1 small turnip, diced
1 medium carrot, diced
1 small potato, diced
1 cup canned diced tomatoes

½ cup cooked or canned
    cannellini beans
½ cup cooked or canned
    chickpeas
½ cup cooked or canned red
    kidney beans
5 cups spring or
    filtered water
1 bay leaf
1 cup cooked small pasta, like
    acini di pepe or elbows
2 sprigs basil, leaves removed
    and shredded

Place oil, garlic and onion in a medium pot over medium heat. When the onion begins to sizzle, add a pinch of salt and a generous pinch of cracked black pepper and sauté until translucent, about 3 minutes. Stir in leek and a pinch of salt and sauté for 1 minute. Stir in celery and a pinch of salt and sauté for 1 minute. Stir in turnip and a pinch of salt and sauté for 1 minute. Stir in carrot and a pinch of salt and sauté for 1 minute. Stir in potato and a pinch of salt and sauté for 1 minute. Stir in tomatoes, beans, water and bay leaf and bring to a boil. Cover and reduce heat to low. Cook until vegetables are quite tender, 30 to 35 minutes. Season with 1 teaspoon salt and simmer for 5 minutes more. Remove and discard bay leaf. Stir in cooked pasta. Serve garnished with basil.

Variation: Vary the veggies and use whatever you have on hand to create a variety of minestrones all your own.

PER SERVING: Calories 169; Protein 7g; Total Fat 1.7g; Saturated Fat .18g; Cholesterol 0mg; Carbohydrate 31.7g; Dietary Fiber 7g; Sodium 833mg

Curried Red Lentil Soup with Cilantro

MAKES 4 TO 5 SERVINGS

1 teaspoon avocado oil

3 cloves fresh garlic, crushed

½ red onion, diced

Sea salt

1 teaspoon curry powder

Generous pinch saffron

1 stalk celery, diced

1 medium carrot, diced

1 cup canned diced tomatoes

1 cup red lentils, rinsed very well

1 bay leaf

4 cups spring or filtered water

2–3 sprigs cilantro, finely minced, for garnish

Heat oil in a medium pot over medium heat. Add garlic, onion and a pinch of salt and sauté until translucent, about 3 minutes. Stir in curry powder. Grind the saffron between your fingers into the onion to release its essence and sauté for 30 seconds. Stir in celery and a pinch of salt and sauté for 1 minute. Stir in carrot and a pinch of salt and sauté for 1 minute. Add tomatoes, lentils, bay leaf and water and bring to a boil. Cover and reduce heat to low. Cook until lentils are quite creamy, about 35 minutes. Season with about 1 teaspoon salt and simmer for 5 to 7 minutes more. Remove and discard bay leaf. Serve garnished with cilantro.

PER SERVING: Calories 203; Protein 14.5g; Total Fat 1.8g; Saturated Fat .22g; Cholesterol 0mg; Carbohydrate 34.5g; Dietary Fiber 16.7g; Sodium 785mg

Miso Soup with Tofu

MAKES 3 TO 4 SERVINGS

½ yellow onion, cut into thin half-moon slices
½ cup fresh daikon, thinly sliced into coins
½ cup shredded green cabbage
½ cup extra-firm tofu, cut into tiny cubes
3 cups spring or filtered water
1½ teaspoons barley or brown rice miso
1–2 scallions, thinly sliced, for garnish

Place all ingredients, except miso and scallions, in a medium pot over medium heat. Bring soup to a boil, cover and reduce heat to low. Cook until daikon is tender, about 7 minutes. Remove a small amount of broth and stir in miso until dissolved. Stir miso mixture into soup and simmer for 3 minutes more. Serve garnished with scallion.

Note: Vary the vegetables to create different versions of miso soup in your diet. Remember, do not boil the miso after adding it to soup. Boiling will destroy the valuable enzymes in the miso that you need.

PER SERVING: Calories 51; Protein 4.2g; Total Fat 2.2g; Saturated Fat .32g; Cholesterol 0mg; Carbohydrate 4.5g; Dietary Fiber 1.2g; Sodium 113mg

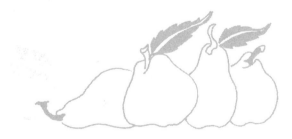

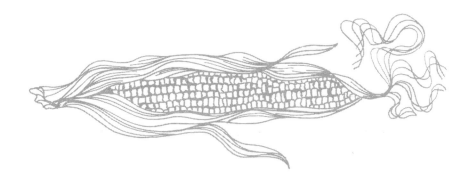

GROOVY GRAINS

We know that our bodies store fat as a reserve, a spare tank to tap into for energy. And fat hangs around, waiting to be used. Carbs, on the other hand, are the preferred energy of your body, with complex carbohydrates—like those found in whole grains—as the premium-grade fuel you need. Composed of long-chain molecules, complex carbs break down more slowly, which nourishes (energizes) you for a longer period of time before hunger sets in again.

But here's the best news about carbohydrates yet. When your body has exhausted its readily available energy resources, it taps into your spare tank of stored energy (that would be fat) for fuel. That's why exercise helps you to lose weight. During exercise, your body burns its carbohydrate stores first and then expends your reserves of fat as energy. Carbs are not the bad guys in dieting. Eating the wrong ones is the problem.

Often referred to as the seeds of life, whole grains supply all the nourishment for the plant. In addition to providing carbohydrates, whole grains supply concentrated amounts of essential nutrients, including fiber, minerals, protein, vitamin E and phytonutrients. Whole grains do it all: B vitamins like pantothenic acid, niacin and B_6 for metabolism, iron for red blood cell formation, zinc for cell repair and fiber for digestion.

Whole grains are not only nourishing and essential to health but they are also yummy. With nutty, satisfying flavors and interesting textures, you won't be bored with your meals once you have added them to your repertoire of recipes. You can mix it up even more and provide variety by choosing from cracked grains as well. Although they are lightly refined, they still provide the lion's share of nutrients you want—and they cook quickly.

Brown Rice and Vegetable Salad

MAKES 4 TO 5 SERVINGS

1 cup short-grain brown rice, rinsed well, soaked for at least 1 hour and up to 8 hours

1½ cups spring or filtered water

Sea salt

1 small zucchini, cut into small dice

2 stalks celery, cut into small dice

1 medium carrot, cut into small dice

1 red bell pepper, roasted (see Note, below), cut into small dice

1 cup baby arugula, coarsely chopped

4 scallions, finely diced

1 shallot, finely diced

Citrusy Mustard Dressing

2 tablespoons fresh lemon juice

¼ cup fresh orange juice

1 tablespoon Dijon mustard

1 tablespoon extra-virgin olive oil

1 teaspoon sea salt

Generous pinch cracked black pepper

Drain rice and discard soaking water. Place rice and water in a pressure cooker and bring to a boil. Add a pinch of salt and seal lid. Bring to full pressure over medium heat. Reduce heat to low and cook rice for 25 minutes. Turn off heat and allow rice to stand in pressure cooker for 25 minutes more. Remove lid and transfer rice to a mixing bowl. (If you do not have a pressure cooker you can boil the rice with 2 parts water to 1 part rice and cook for 50 minutes or until all liquid is absorbed.)

Stir the vegetables into the hot rice so they cook just a tiny bit. They should be digestible but still crunchy.

Make dressing: Whisk all ingredients together in a small bowl, adjusting the salt and pepper to your taste.

Stir the dressing into the hot rice mixture to coat. Serve warm or at room temperature.

Note: Soaking brown rice before cooking helps to rid it of a substance called phytic acid, which can inhibit your body's ability to efficiently use calcium.

Note: To roast a pepper, place whole bell pepper over an open flame. Using tongs, carefully turn the bell pepper until it is completely charred and blackened. Remove from heat and place in a paper sack. Fold the top of the sack over to seal and let the pepper steam for 10 minutes. Remove the pepper and peel the charred skin away. You may also buy roasted peppers in a jar at the market.

PER SERVING: Calories 244; Protein 5.7g; Total Fat 5g; Saturated Fat .55g; Cholesterol 0mg; Carbohydrate 45.2g; Dietary Fiber 4.2g; Sodium 733mg

Polenta with Spicy Sauteed Broccoli Rabe

MAKES 4 TO 5 SERVINGS

Polenta
1 cup corn grits
5 cups spring or filtered water
Pinch sea salt
1 teaspoon unsweetened almond milk

Spicy Sauteed Broccoli Rabe
2 teaspoons extra-virgin olive oil
2 cloves fresh garlic, finely minced
½ red onion, cut into small dice
Generous pinch crushed red pepper flakes
1 red bell pepper, roasted (see Note, page 153), thinly sliced into ribbons
1 large bunch broccoli rabe, rinsed well, tips of stems removed and stems
    cut into bite-size pieces

Make the polenta: Place grits, water and salt in a saucepan and whisk well. Place pan over medium heat and whisk until the mixture boils. Reduce heat to low and cook, whisking frequently, until the mixture "heaves," meaning a big bubble bursts at the center of the polenta. Remove from heat and whisk in almond milk. Spoon polenta into a pie plate and set aside. It will set firmly in about 30 minutes. You may also serve it soft, but you must time it so it can be served immediately for that to work out.

Make the broccoli rabe: Prepare the broccoli rabe when the polenta is about 80% done cooking if you are serving it soft, or when it's firmly set, depending on which way you are serving it. Place oil, garlic and onion in a skillet over medium heat. When the onion begins to sizzle, add a pinch of salt and red pepper flakes and sauté until onion is translucent, about 3 minutes. Stir in bell pepper and a pinch of salt and sauté for 1 minute. Stir broccoli rabe into skillet, with ½ teaspoon salt and sauté just until rabe is wilted and bright green, about 4 minutes. Transfer to a serving bowl.

To serve, cut polenta into wedges or spoon soft portions into bowls. Top with rabe mixture and serve hot.

PER SERVING: Calories 78; Protein 2.5g; Total Fat 2.5g; Saturated Fat .36g; Cholesterol 0mg; Carbohydrate 12.2g; Dietary Fiber .57g; Sodium 403mg

Farro Salad with Peas, Arugula and Tomatoes
MAKES 2 SERVINGS

1 clove fresh garlic, crushed
¼ red onion, cut into small dice
½ cup farro, rinsed well
1 cup spring or filtered water
Sea salt
½ cup fresh or frozen petite peas
8–10 cherry tomatoes, quartered
1 cup baby arugula
2 teaspoons extra-virgin olive oil
Generous pinch cracked black pepper
2 tablespoons fresh lemon juice

Place garlic, onion, farro and water in a saucepan and bring to a boil over medium heat. Add a pinch of salt, cover and reduce heat to low. Cook until grain is tender and all the water has been absorbed, 25 to 30 minutes. While the farro is hot, stir in remaining ingredients and ½ teaspoon salt as the final seasoning. Transfer to a serving bowl and serve warm or at room temperature.

PER SERVING: Calories 186; Protein 6g; Total Fat 5.1g; Saturated Fat .72g; Cholesterol 0mg; Carbohydrate 30.9g; Dietary Fiber 5.8g; Sodium 627mg

Millet with Cinnamon Onions

MAKES 4 TO 5 SERVINGS

Cinnamon Onions
3 red onions, each cut into 8 wedges
2 teaspoons extra-virgin olive oil
⅔ teaspoon sea salt
½ teaspoon ground cinnamon
1 teaspoon brown rice syrup

Millet
1 cup millet
3 cups spring or filtered water
Pinch sea salt
Scant pinch nutmeg
2 to 3 sprigs fresh flat-leaf parsley, finely minced, for garnish

Make onions: Preheat oven to 375 degrees. Place onion wedges in a large bowl and mix with all other ingredients until coated. Arrange in a shallow rimmed baking sheet, avoiding overlap. Cover tightly with foil and bake for 45 minutes. Remove foil and return onions to oven for about 10 minutes, until slightly browned.

Make millet: Begin making the millet when onions have been cooking for 25 minutes. Place millet and water in a saucepan and bring to a boil over medium heat. Add salt and nutmeg; cover and reduce heat to low. Cook until millet is soft and the water has been absorbed, about 30 minutes. Stir in parsley. Transfer millet to a shallow serving bowl and spoon onions over top. Serve immediately.

PER SERVING: Calories 246; Protein 6.4g; Total Fat 4.5g; Saturated Fat .71g; Cholesterol 0mg; Carbohydrate 44.7g; Dietary Fiber 5.8g; Sodium 419mg

Quinoa Tabbouleh with Avocado

MAKES 4 TO 5 SERVINGS

1 cup quinoa, rinsed very well (see Note, below)

2 cups spring or filtered water

Sea salt

Cracked black pepper

2 tablespoons fresh lemon juice

2 teaspoons extra-virgin olive oil

½ teaspoon brown rice syrup

6–7 sprigs flat-leaf parsley, coarsely chopped (about ⅓ cup)

2 cloves fresh garlic, very finely minced

½ red bell pepper, roasted (see Note, page 153), cut into small dice

¼ red onion, cut into small dice

2–3 plum tomatoes, seeded, cut into small dice

½ cup small dice cucumber

½ avocado, ripe but firm, cut into small dice

Add quinoa and water to a saucepan and bring to a boil over medium heat. Add a pinch of salt; cover and reduce heat to low. Cook until quinoa has absorbed all the water and has opened (a small "tail" forms on each grain, like a tadpole), about 25 minutes. Transfer quinoa to a mixing bowl, fluff with a fork and allow to come to room temperature.

While the quinoa cools, whisk together ½ teaspoon sea salt, ⅛ teaspoon black pepper, lemon juice, oil and rice syrup. Set aside.

When the quinoa is cooled, fold in oil mixture and all the vegetables, tossing very gently to incorporate. Do not break the avocado into mush. Serve within 2 hours of making this dish or it will get soggy. (If making ahead, do not add the oil mixture until close to serving time.)

Note: It is important to wash quinoa very well, as it is coated with an oily substance called saponin that can make it taste bitter.

PER SERVING: Calories 241; Protein 6.7g; Total Fat 8.8g; Saturated Fat 1.2g; Cholesterol 0mg; Carbohydrate 35.6g; Dietary Fiber 4.7g; Sodium 337mg

Basmati Rice with Curried Vegetables

MAKES 5 TO 6 SERVINGS

1 cup brown basmati rice, rinsed well, soaked for at least 1 hour and up to
    8 hours
1½ cups spring or filtered water
Sea salt
2 teaspoons avocado oil
½ yellow onion, cut into small dice
3 cloves fresh garlic, crushed
1 tablespoon finely minced fresh ginger
1 teaspoon curry powder
1 small carrot, cut into small dice
2 red potatoes, cut into small dice
1 medium zucchini, cut into small dice
1 cup small cauliflower florets
2 teaspoons finely minced fresh cilantro
2 teaspoons chia seeds (see Note, below)

Drain rice, discarding soaking water. Place rice and water in a pressure cooker over medium heat. When rice boils, add a pinch of salt; seal the lid and bring to full pressure. Reduce heat to low and cook for 25 minutes. Turn off heat and allow pressure cooker to stand undisturbed for another 25 minutes.

While rice is standing, place avocado oil in a deep skillet over medium heat. Add onion, garlic, ginger, curry powder and a pinch of salt and sauté until onion is translucent, about 3 minutes. Stir in carrot and a pinch of salt and sauté for 1 minute. Stir in potatoes and a pinch of salt and sauté for 1 minute. Stir in zucchini and a pinch of salt and sauté for 1 minute. Stir in cauliflower and a pinch of salt and sauté for 1 minute. Add 3 to 4 tablespoons of water; cover and steam vegetables until the potatoes are just tender, but not mushy, 5 to 6 minutes.

Transfer rice to a serving bowl and gently fold curried vegetables and cilantro into hot rice. Serve garnished with a sprinkle of chia seeds.

Note: Tiny chia seeds, found in natural food stores, are rich sources of omega-3 fatty acids, fiber, iron and other nutrients.

PER SERVING: Calorie 223; Protein 5.8g; Total Fat 3.9g; Saturated Fat .8g; Cholesterol 0mg; Carbohydrate 45.8g; Dietary Fiber 4.8g; Sodium 173mg

Quinoa and Sweet Potato Croquettes with Black Bean Salsa

MAKES ABOUT 6 SERVINGS

Black Bean Salsa

½ red onion, cut into small dice

2 plum tomatoes, seeded, cut into small dice

1 small jalapeño chile, finely minced

1 clove fresh garlic, finely minced

¼ teaspoon sea salt

1 cup cooked or canned black beans

3 scallions, finely minced

1 tablespoon fresh lemon or lime juice

1 teaspoon extra-virgin olive oil

Quinoa and Sweet Potato Croquettes

2 cups spring or filtered water

1 small sweet potato, peeled, diced

1 cup quinoa, rinsed very well

Sea salt

1 teaspoon extra-virgin olive oil

3 scallions, finely diced

4 sprigs parsley, minced

1 jalapeño chile, seeded, finely minced

½ teaspoon ground cumin

½ teaspoon dried oregano

2 cloves fresh garlic, finely minced

½ cup pureed silken tofu

3 tablespoons grated vegan mozzarella cheese alternative

Avocado oil, for frying

Whole wheat bread crumbs, for coating croquettes

Make the salsa: Combine all ingredients in a small bowl. Mix well, cover and set aside for flavors to develop.

Make the croquettes: Bring water to a boil and add sweet potato and quinoa. Add a pinch of salt; cover and bring to a boil. Reduce heat to low and cook until quinoa has absorbed the water and has opened, about 20 minutes.

While the quinoa cooks, place olive oil in a skillet over medium heat. Add scallions, parsley, chile, cumin, oregano and garlic and sauté for 1 to 2 minutes. Transfer to a mixing bowl.

Mash cooked sweet potato and quinoa together with a fork to break up the sweet potato. Fold in scallion mixture, tofu and cheese alternative. Mix very well. Form quinoa mixture into 2-inch patties.

Heat 1 tablespoon of avocado oil in a skillet over medium heat, turning the skillet so that the oils coats the surface. Dredge croquettes in bread crumbs to coat. Fry until golden on each side, turning once to ensure even browning, about 2 minutes per side. Transfer to a platter and spoon 1 to 2 tablespoons salsa on top of each croquette.

PER SERVING: Calorie 223; Protein 8.1g; Total Fat 6.7g; Saturated Fat .89g; Cholesterol 0mg; Carbohydrate 35.3g; Dietary Fiber 5.2g; Sodium 337mg

Penne with Pan-Roasted Tomato and Chile Sauce
MAKES 4 SERVINGS

Pan-Roasted Tomato and Chile Sauce
2 pounds ripe plum tomatoes
3 serrano chiles, seeded, stems removed
2 teaspoons extra-virgin olive oil
3 cloves fresh garlic, crushed
½ red onion, cut into small dice
1½ teaspoons sea salt
Generous pinch crushed red pepper flakes
⅛ teaspoon cracked black pepper

Sea salt
Extra-virgin olive oil

2 cups whole wheat penne

2 tablespoons coarsely chopped fresh flat-leaf parsley

2 tablespoons coarsely chopped fresh basil

Make the sauce: Line a large skillet with foil. Arrange tomatoes and chiles in the skillet and cook over medium heat, turning occasionally, until the skins blister and begin to blacken in spots, about 20 minutes for the tomatoes, 10 minutes for the chiles. Remove from heat and cool the tomatoes just enough to be able to handle them. Peel the skins from the tomatoes and chiles and coarsely chop them together. Transfer to a mixing bowl and set aside.

Place oil, garlic and onion in a deep skillet over medium heat. When the onion begins to sizzle, add a pinch of the salt, red pepper flakes and black pepper. Sauté until the onion is translucent, about 3 minutes. Stir in tomato mixture and add the remaining salt. Reduce heat to low and simmer for 10 to 15 minutes.

While the sauce cooks, bring a pot of water to a boil with a generous pinch of salt and a splash of olive oil. When the water boils, add penne and cook al dente, about 8 minutes. Using a slotted spoon, transfer the penne to the sauce in the skillet. Add parsley and basil and stir until the penne is coated with sauce. Serve immediately.

PER SERVING: Calories 262; Protein 10g; Total Fat 3.8g; Saturated Fat .57g; Cholesterol 0mg; Carbohydrate 52.3g; Dietary Fiber 7.2g; Sodium 888mg

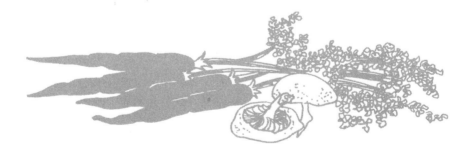

Linguine al Verde

MAKES 4 SERVINGS; 3 CUPS SAUCE

Verde Sauce
3 cups loosely packed fresh basil leaves
3 cups loosely packed fresh flat-leaf parsley leaves
10 scallions, coarsely chopped
5 cloves fresh garlic, peeled, left whole
Grated zest of 1 lemon
Juice of ½ orange
3 ounces capers, drained well
5 pitted green olives, drained well
1 tablespoon sweet white miso
Generous pinch crushed red pepper flakes
⅓–½ cup extra-virgin olive oil

6–8 ounces whole wheat linguine
4–5 cherry tomatoes, quartered, for garnish

Make Verde Sauce: Place basil, parsley, scallions, garlic, lemon zest and orange juice in a food processor and pulse to chop ingredients. Add capers, olives, miso and red pepper flakes and pulse to combine. With the motor running, slowly add olive oil until you have a thick, creamy consistency. Do not make this too liquidy or the sauce will not stick to the linguine. Reserve ½ cup of the sauce. Freeze the remaining sauce in either ½-cup or 1-cup containers. One cup coats 1 pound of pasta.

Cook linguine al dente in boiling salted water; drain, but do not rinse. Toss hot pasta with the reserved ½ cup sauce. Serve garnished with cherry tomatoes.

PER SERVING: Calories 306; Protein 8.7g; Total Fat 14.1g; Saturated Fat 1.9g; Cholesterol 0mg; Carbohydrate 40.1g; Dietary Fiber 5.8g; Sodium 489mg

Orecchiette with Green Olive Pesto

MAKES 4 SERVINGS

Green Olive Pesto
2 cloves fresh garlic, peeled, left whole
1 shallot, coarsely chopped
¼ cup pitted green olives (Niçoise are best)
¼ cup loosely packed fresh flat-leaf parsley leaves
¼ cup loosely packed fresh basil leaves
¼ cup extra-virgin olive oil

8 oil-cured black olives, pitted, very finely minced
½ teaspoon sea salt
2 plum tomatoes, seeded, finely chopped
2 cups orecchiette, cooked al dente, ¼ cup pasta cooking water reserved
4 basil sprigs, for garnish

Make pesto: Combine garlic, shallot, green olives, parsley and basil in a food processor. Pulse to coarsely chop. With the motor running, slowly add olive oil and process until fully incorporated into the olive mixture, but do not overprocess. This should be a coarse pesto, not smooth.

Heat a deep skillet over medium heat and add pesto, black olives, salt and tomatoes. Cook, stirring constantly, for 2 minutes. Stir in orecchiette and pasta cooking water and cook, stirring, until the water is absorbed, about 2 minutes more. Serve hot, garnished with basil sprigs.

PER SERVING: Calories 251; Protein 3.3g; Total Fat 17.7g; Saturated Fat 2g; Cholesterol 0mg; Carbohydrate 20.4g; Dietary Fiber 1.36g; Sodium 532mg

Fried Soba with Ginger and Scallion
MAKES 3 SERVINGS

2 teaspoons avocado oil, plus extra for cooking noodles

8 ounces soba noodles

2 tablespoons finely minced fresh ginger

1 bunch scallions, thinly sliced on the diagonal

1 tablespoon natural shoyu

1 teaspoon brown rice syrup

Bring a pot of water and a splash of avocado oil to a boil. When the water boils, cook soba until 80% done, about 7 minutes. Drain and rinse very well. Set aside.

Heat the 2 teaspoons oil in a skillet over medium heat. Add ginger, scallions and a splash of shoyu and sauté until scallions wilt, about 3 minutes. Place noodles on top of cooked scallions, season with remaining shoyu and drizzle with rice syrup. Cover, reduce heat to low and simmer for 3 minutes. Stir well and serve hot.

PER SERVING: Calories 305; Protein 11.1g; Total Fat 3.75g; Saturated Fat .48g; Cholesterol 0mg; Carbohydrate 61.5g; Dietary Fiber 1.1g; Sodium 910mg

Garlic-Scented Kasha Pilaf
MAKES 4 SERVINGS

½ cup kasha

2 teaspoons extra-virgin olive oil

2 cloves fresh garlic, crushed

½ red onion, cut into small dice

½ teaspoon sea salt

Scant pinch cracked black pepper

1 stalk celery, cut into small dice

1 medium carrot, cut into small dice

1½ cups spring or filtered water

3 tablespoons pine nuts

2 teaspoons chia seeds

Place kasha in a dry skillet and pan-toast it over medium-low heat, stirring constantly until fragrant, about 3 minutes. Transfer to a bowl and set aside.

Place oil, garlic and onion in a saucepan over medium heat. When the onion begins to sizzle, add a pinch of the salt and pepper and sauté until translucent, about 3 minutes. Stir in celery and a pinch of the salt and sauté for 1 minute. Stir in carrot and a pinch of the salt and sauté for 1 minute. Stir in kasha and cook, stirring, for 1 minute. Add water, cover and bring to a boil. Add remaining salt; reduce heat to low and cook, stirring occasionally, until the water has been absorbed, about 10 minutes. Remove from heat and allow kasha to stand, undisturbed in the pan, for 5 minutes. Fluff with a fork and transfer to a serving bowl. Serve garnished with pine nuts and chia seeds.

PER SERVING: Calories 130; Protein 4.7g; Total Fat 4.3g; Saturated Fat .8g; Cholesterol 0mg; Carbohydrate 20.6g; Dietary Fiber 3.7g; Sodium 305mg

Amaranth and Corn
MAKES 2 TO 3 SERVINGS

1¼ cups spring or filtered water

½ cup amaranth

¼ cup fresh or frozen corn kernels

Pinch sea salt

1 teaspoon chia seeds

Bring water to a boil in a saucepan over medium heat. Whisk in amaranth and cook, stirring constantly, until mixture returns to a boil. Add corn and salt and cook, stirring occasionally, until the water has been absorbed and the amaranth is smooth and creamy, 20 to 25 minutes. Serve immediately with a sprinkle of chia seeds.

PER SERVING: Calories 208; Protein 7.9g; Total Fat 3.7g; Saturated Fat 1g; Cholesterol 0mg; Carbohydrate 37.3g; Dietary Fiber 8.3g; Sodium 80mg

Citrus-Scented Seeded Muffins

MAKES 24 MINI MUFFINS

1½ cups whole wheat pastry flour
½ cup semolina flour
1 teaspoon baking powder
1 teaspoon baking soda
¼ teaspoon sea salt
⅓ cup avocado oil
3 tablespoons brown rice syrup
½ cup erythritol
    (see Note, below)
Grated zest of 1 lemon
Grated zest of 1 orange

½ cup combined lemon and
   orange juice
1 teaspoon pure vanilla extract
⅔–1 cup unsweetened almond
   milk
1 teaspoon chia seeds
2 teaspoons chopped
sunflower seeds
2 teaspoons chopped
pumpkin seeds

Preheat oven to 350 degrees. Lightly oil a 24-cup mini muffin pan.

Whisk together flours, baking powder, baking soda and salt. Combine oil, rice syrup and erythritol in a small saucepan and cook, stirring, until the granules dissolve, 2 to 3 minutes. Remove from heat and whisk in zests, juices and vanilla. Mix into dry ingredients and slowly mix in almond milk until a smooth batter forms. Fold in seeds until incorporated through the batter. Divide batter evenly among muffin cups, filling cups two-thirds full.

Bake for 20 to 25 minutes, until the tops of the muffins spring back to the touch. Cool for 5 minutes before carefully removing the muffins from the cups. Transfer to a cooling rack and cool completely. (You can freeze and thaw these in pairs so you won't be tempted to eat the whole batch.)

Note: Erythritol is a natural no-calorie sweetener made from fermented sugar alcohol. Completely natural, this sweetener is about 75% as sweet as sugar but without the calories. It is available at natural food stores and online.

PER MUFFIN: Calories 67; Protein 1.3g; Total Fat 3.4g; Saturated Fat .41g; Cholesterol 0mg; Carbohydrate 8.1g; Dietary Fiber .87g; Sodium 94mg

Chili-Spiced Cornbread

MAKES 9 PIECES

1 cup yellow cornmeal

1 cup whole wheat pastry flour

1 teaspoon baking powder

1 teaspoon baking soda

1 teaspoon chili powder

¼ teaspoon sea salt

1 tablespoon brown rice syrup

1 teaspoon brown rice vinegar

1 cup unsweetened almond milk

Preheat oven to 350 degrees. Lightly oil a 9-inch-square baking pan.

Whisk cornmeal, flour, baking powder, baking soda, chili powder and sea salt in a mixing bowl. Whisk rice syrup, rice vinegar and almond milk together in another bowl. Mix wet ingredients into the dry ingredients to form a smooth batter. Spoon into prepared pan and bake for 30 to 35 minutes, until the center of the cornbread springs back to the touch. Cool for 10 minutes before cutting into squares.

PER PIECE: Calories 97; Protein 2.7g; Total Fat .8g; Saturated Fat .04g; Cholesterol 0mg; Carbohydrate 20.8g; Dietary Fiber 2.24g; Sodium 256mg

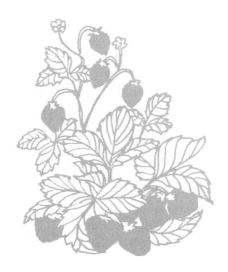

Better French Toast with Fruit Salsa

MAKES 2 SERVINGS

Fruit Salsa

1 cup strawberries, tops removed

1 Granny Smith apple

1 kiwifruit, peeled

2 teaspoons brown rice syrup

1 tablespoon fresh orange juice

Pinch sea salt

Scant pinch ground cinnamon

French Toast

2 very ripe bananas

¼ cup almond milk

1 teaspoon pure vanilla extract

Generous pinch ground cinnamon

Pinch sea salt

¼ cup spring or filtered water

2 tablespoons avocado oil

4 slices whole grain bread

Make the salsa: Pulse all the fruit in a food processor until coarsely chopped. Whisk together rice syrup, orange juice, salt and cinnamon. Toss with fruit and set aside to allow flavors to develop.

Make French toast: Place bananas, almond milk, vanilla, cinnamon, salt and water in a blender or food processor and puree until smooth and the consistency of beaten eggs.

Heat avocado oil in a skillet or griddle pan over medium heat. Dredge bread in banana mixture on both sides and lay on griddle pan. Cook until browned on both sides, turning once, about 2 minutes per side.

Arrange 2 slices of French toast on each plate and ladle fruit salsa over top.

Note: On the days I indulge in this breakfast, I usually only eat 2 meals and a snack to watch my calorie intake.

PER SERVING: Calories 452; Protein 6.5g; Total Fat 16.1g; Saturated Fat 1.89g; Cholesterol 0mg; Carbohydrate 78.8g; Dietary Fiber 17.3g; Sodium 328mg

Tortillas with Black Bean Sauce

MAKES 4 SERVINGS

Black Bean Sauce

2 teaspoons avocado oil

2 cloves fresh garlic, crushed

½ red onion, cut into thin half-moon slices

Sea salt

Generous pinch crushed red pepper flakes

6 maitake mushrooms, soaked until tender, thinly sliced

1 red bell pepper, roasted (see Note, page 153), thinly sliced into ribbons

1 medium zucchini, cut into fine matchstick pieces

1 yellow summer squash, cut into fine matchstick pieces

1 cup cooked or canned black beans, mashed with a fork

¼ cup white wine

1 tablespoon natural soy sauce

2 teaspoons brown rice syrup

2 tablespoons arrowroot dissolved in 2 tablespoons water

4 whole wheat tortillas

2 cups baby arugula

Make Black Bean Sauce: Heat oil in a deep skillet over medium heat. Add garlic, onion, a pinch of sea salt and red pepper flakes and sauté until onion is translucent, about 3 minutes. Stir in mushrooms and a pinch of salt and sauté for 1 minute. Stir in bell pepper and a pinch of salt and sauté for 1 minute. Stir in zucchini and a pinch of salt and sauté for 1 minute. Stir in squash and a pinch of salt and sauté for 1 minute. Stir in beans, wine, soy sauce and rice syrup and cook, stirring, for about 3 minutes. Stir arrowroot mixture into bean mixture. Stir until the arrowroot is clear and mixture thickens slightly.

To serve, lay tortillas on individual plates. Stir arugula into hot bean mixture to wilt it. Spoon equal amounts of black bean sauce on each tortilla, roll and serve.

PER SERVING: Calories 240; Protein 8.1g; Total Fat 4.1g; Saturated Fat .33g; Cholesterol 0mg; Carbohydrate 45.4g; Dietary Fiber 6.89g; Sodium 777mg

Buckwheat Pancakes with Red Chili Syrup

MAKES 6 PANCAKES; 3 (2-PANCAKE) SERVINGS

½ cup buckwheat flour
½ cup whole wheat pastry flour
1 teaspoon baking powder
1 teaspoon baking soda
Generous pinch sea salt
Generous pinch ground cinnamon
1 tablespoon apple cider vinegar
I cup unsweetened almond milk
Red Chili Syrup (below)

Place a lightly oiled griddle or flat-bottomed skillet over medium heat.
Make the batter: Whisk together flours, baking powder, baking soda, salt and cinnamon. Whisk together vinegar and almond milk and mix into the dry ingredients, whisking briskly to incorporate the ingredients fully.

Spoon batter in ¼-cup scoops onto hot griddle. Cook until the edges bubble and are lightly browned, 2 to 3 minutes. Flip and cook the other sides until the pancakes are solid and well done, 2 to 3 minutes. Serve with Red Chili Syrup.

PER PANCAKE: Calories 68; Protein 2.3g; Total Fat .44g; Saturated Fat .07g; Cholesterol 0mg; Carbohydrate 13.8g; Dietary Fiber 1.76g; Sodium 330mg

Red Chili Syrup

MAKES 4 SERVINGS

½ cup brown rice syrup
2 teaspoons pomegranate juice
½ teaspoon chili powder
Pinch sea salt

Place all ingredients in a small saucepan over low heat. Simmer, stirring constantly, for 3 to 4 minutes to develop flavors.

PER SERVING: Calories 65; Protein 0g; Total Fat 0g; Saturated Fat 0g; Cholesterol 0mg; Carbohydrate 21g; Dietary Fiber 0g; Sodium 35mg

hour. Allow pressure to reduce naturally, open the lid, stir cereal and serve hot.

Variations: Add ¼ cup fresh or frozen corn kernels, ¼ cup diced winter squash or carrot and cook with the grain. Or sprinkle the cooked cereal with toasted sesame seeds or chia seeds.

If sweet taste is what you crave on some mornings, cook a few raisins or chopped apples or pears in with the grain for a bit of delicate sweetness that will satisfy you and still keep you level.

PER SERVING: Calories 115; Protein 2.47g; Total Fat 1.22g; Saturated Fat .29g; Cholesterol 0mg; Carbohydrate 25.1g; Dietary Fiber 1.54g; Sodium 48mg

Quick Breakfast Porridge

This for a quicker breakfast made from leftover cooked grains and quick-cooking whole grains. You can also make variations of this dish the same as Hearty Grain Breakfast Porridge (page 172).

MAKES 3 SERVINGS

1 cup leftover cooked grain (brown rice, millet, kasha, quinoa or other grain)
Spring or filtered water
Pinch sea salt

Place grain in a saucepan. Add water to just cover the grain and soak overnight. In the morning, add salt and bring to a boil. Cover, reduce heat to low and cook until the liquid is absorbed and the grain is quite soft, about 20 minutes.

PER SERVING: Calories 115; Protein 2.47g; Total Fat 1.22g; Saturated Fat .29g; Cholesterol 0mg; Carbohydrate 25.1g; Dietary Fiber 1.54g; Sodium 48mg

Light Grain Porridge

Using lighter grains gives you a hot breakfast in minutes.

MAKES 2 SERVINGS

½ cup quinoa, amaranth, kasha, couscous, bulgur or teff
1 cup spring or filtered water
Pinch sea salt

Place grain and water in a saucepan and bring to a boil. Add salt, cover and reduce heat to low. Cook until the liquid is absorbed, 15 to 20 minutes. The exception is couscous, which cooks in 5 minutes.

Variations: All of these grains love pairing up with corn kernels, so enjoy that bit of sweetness. A sprinkling of chia seeds over the cooked cereal will ensure you get your omega-3 fatty acids for the day.

PER SERVING: Calories 159; Protein 5.57g; Total Fat 2.5g; Saturated Fat .25g; Cholesterol 0mg; Carbohydrate 29.2g; Dietary Fiber 2.5g; Sodium 78mg

Polenta Breakfast Porridge

This fast dish uses corn meal or grits, but you can use this recipe with any cracked grain you wish.

MAKES 3 SERVINGS

½ cup corn grits or meal
2½ cups spring or filtered water
Pinch sea salt
Pinch dried basil

Combine all ingredients in a saucepan over medium heat. Cook, whisking, until mixture comes to a boil. Reduce heat to low and cook, whisking frequently, until mixture bubbles in the center, 20 to 25 minutes. Serve hot.

PER SERVING: Calories 24; Protein .56g; Total Fat .08g; Saturated Fat .01g; Cholesterol 0mg; Carbohydrate 5.24g; Dietary Fiber 0g; Sodium 46mg

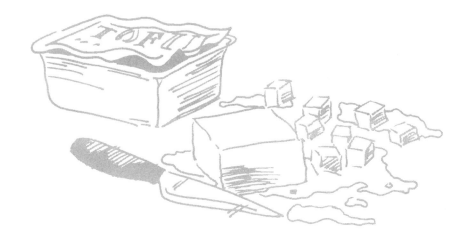

THE MAIN EVENT

Americans love a main course. For many of you, it's not a meal unless there's a slab of meat in the center of your plate with a few steamed baby carrots on the side for garnish. It's our culture; it's how you think of meals. Well, as the saying goes, "Them days are over!"

Vegan eating is different than conventional approaches to meat-structured meals. In whole-foods vegan eating, we are less about a centerpiece dish surrounded by sides and more about bringing together a varying number of ingredients to compose a beautiful, delicious plate of balanced nutrients, sheathed in a variety of textures and flavors. It's that simple.

But because I love you and because I want you to be happy, I am including this chapter comprising beans and soy foods as the "main courses" of the meal. If meat is the current main attraction on your plate, then use beans and bean by-products, the vegan sources of protein, as your new one—anything to make the rethinking part a bit easier.

After a month or so of skipping the beef and instead getting the protein you need from vegetable sources, you will be stunned at how strong and vital you feel, how light and energized. Lethargy and fogginess will be a thing of the past. You'll wonder why you waited so long to say, "Hold the meat, please."

Dr. Dean Ornish said it best: "I don't understand why asking people to eat a well-balanced vegetarian diet is considered drastic, while it is medically conservative to cut people open and put them on cholesterol-lowering drugs for the rest of their lives."

I bet tofu seems more appealing now.

Creamy Minted White Beans
MAKES 4 TO 5 SERVINGS

1 cup dried cannellini beans, rinsed well, soaked in hot water for 1 hour
    (see Note, page 177)

3 cups spring or filtered water

1 bay leaf

1 tablespoon extra-virgin olive oil

2 cloves fresh garlic, crushed

2 shallots, minced

Sea salt

Generous pinch cracked black pepper

1 red bell pepper, roasted (see Note, page 153), cut into small dice

8 artichoke hearts, quartered (see Note, page 177)

¼ cup dry white wine

¼ cup coarsely chopped fresh flat-leaf parsley

½ cup coarsely chopped fresh mint

2 tablespoons fresh lemon juice

Drain beans and discard soaking water. Place beans, water and bay leaf in a saucepan over medium heat. When the beans come to a boil, cover and reduce heat to low. Cook until the beans are just tender, about 45 minutes to 1 hour.

When the beans are just about ready, place oil, garlic and shallots in a deep skillet over medium heat. When the shallots begin to sizzle, add a pinch of salt and black pepper and sauté until the shallots are just beginning to brown, about 7 minutes. Stir in bell pepper, artichokes and a pinch of salt and sauté for 2 minutes. Add wine, reduce heat to low and simmer, uncovered, until the wine is absorbed and begins to deglaze into a syrup, about 5 minutes. Stir in beans, 1 teaspoon salt, parsley and mint and cook, stirring, until the herbs wilt and turn bright green, about 1 minute. Remove from heat and stir in lemon juice. Serve hot.

Note: Soaking beans is not necessary and actually robs them of valuable enzymes, but you can soak them for 1 hour to shorten your cooking time slightly. To save even more time, use canned organic beans instead of cooking them from scratch. Canned beans will not give you the same vitality and energy as cooking them will, but in a pinch, they can do the job. Just rinse them very well before use to remove the stale water and excess salt from the can.

Note: Artichoke hearts can be purchased in jars or cans. Be sure to buy the ones that are not marinated in oil; you may not want the calories or the flavor. Also, you can take fresh artichokes down to their hearts by simply cutting away the outer leaves and removing the chokes.

PER SERVING: Calories 244; Protein 13.7g; Total Fat 4g; Saturated Fat .63g; Cholesterol 0mg; Carbohydrate 38.1g; Dietary Fiber 9.7g; Sodium 831mg

Moroccan Lentil Stew

MAKES 5 TO 6 SERVINGS

2 teaspoons extra-virgin olive oil	1½ cups ½-inch cubes butternut
2 cloves fresh garlic, finely minced	squash
2 teaspoons finely minced ginger	1½ cups ½-inch cubes sweet potato
½ red onion, cut into chunks	1 cup canned diced tomatoes
Sea salt	1 cup green or brown lentils, rinsed
1 teaspoon curry powder	very well
½ teaspoon ground cinnamon	1 bay leaf
½ teaspoon ground cumin	3 cups spring or filtered water
Generous pinch cardamom	2 cups fresh or frozen petite peas
Generous pinch cayenne pepper	

Place oil, garlic, ginger and onion in a heavy saucepan over medium heat. When the onion begins to sizzle, add a pinch of salt, curry powder, cinnamon, cumin, cardamom and cayenne and sauté for about 3 minutes. Stir in squash and a pinch of salt and sauté for 1 minute. Stir in sweet potato and a pinch of salt and sauté for 1 minute. Add tomatoes, lentils, bay leaf and water. Bring to a boil, cover and reduce heat to low. Cook until lentils are soft and the water has been absorbed, creating a thick stew, about 45 minutes. Season with 1 teaspoon salt and stir in peas. Cook for 2 minutes to cook peas through. Serve hot.

PER SERVING: Calories 262; Protein 15.6g; Total Fat 2.7g; Saturated Fat .39g; Cholesterol 0mg; Carbohydrate 46.6g; Dietary Fiber 18.7g; Sodium 672mg

Braised Tofu with Spring Greens and Pineapple-Curry Vinaigrette

MAKES 2 SERVINGS

Pineapple-Curry Vinaigrette
3 tablespoons extra-virgin olive oil
1 teaspoon curry powder
½ teaspoon ground cumin
½ teaspoon sea salt
Cracked black pepper
¼ cup fresh pineapple juice
2 tablespoons red wine vinegar
3 scallions, finely minced

Braised Tofu
2 teaspoons avocado oil
2 teaspoons soy sauce
2 teaspoons brown rice syrup
½ teaspoon curry powder
Scant pinch chili powder
8 ounces extra-firm tofu, cut into 6 slices

Spring Greens
2 cups organic baby spring greens
1 small cucumber, cut into fine julienne pieces
⅓ cup fine julienne pieces fresh daikon

Make the vinaigrette: Place oil, curry powder, cumin, salt and pepper in a small skillet and cook, stirring, over low heat until fragrant, about 2 minutes. This brings out the curry powder's heat. Remove from heat and whisk in remaining ingredients. Set aside to cool and to allow flavors to develop.

Make the tofu: Combine oil, soy sauce, syrup, curry powder and chili powder in a saucepan over medium heat. Stir to combine ingredients. When the oil is hot, pat tofu slices dry with a kitchen towel and arrange them in the hot oil. Cook until browned, 2 to 3 minutes. Turn and brown on the other side.

While the tofu cooks, prepare the salad greens: Combine greens with cucumber and daikon in a large bowl. Toss with vinaigrette to coat and arrange salad on a shallow platter. Arrange tofu slices on top and serve immediately.

PER SERVING: Calories 375; Protein 11.6g; Total Fat 31.7g; Saturated Fat 4.38g; Cholesterol 0mg; Carbohydrate 14.8g; Dietary Fiber 3.6g; Sodium 911mg

White Beans with Sage and Olive Oil
MAKES 2 SERVINGS

1 tablespoon extra-virgin olive oil
2 cloves fresh garlic, crushed
½ red onion, cut into small dice
Sea salt
½ cup coarsely chopped fresh sage
Scant pinch cracked black pepper
1 cup cooked or canned cannellini beans
¼ cup white wine
2 tablespoons fresh lemon juice
3–4 fresh sage leaves, for garnish

Place oil, garlic and onion in a skillet over medium heat. When the onion sizzles, add a pinch of salt and sauté until translucent, about 3 minutes. Add chopped sage, pepper, beans, wine and ½ teaspoon salt. Reduce heat to low and simmer until beans are heated through and the wine has deglazed a bit, 5 minutes. Remove from heat and add lemon juice. Stir well and serve garnished with fresh sage leaves.

Note: You can use canned organic beans in this recipe. Just rinse them well before use. Or you can cook ½ cup dried beans with 1½ cups of water for about 1 hour. It will yield about 1 cup cooked beans.

PER SERVING: Calories 265; Protein 10.4g; Total Fat 7.8g; Saturated Fat 1.1g; Cholesterol 0mg; Carbohydrate 34.9g; Dietary Fiber 6.9g; Sodium 585mg

Pan-Braised Tempeh with Tropical Salsa
MAKES 4 SERVINGS

Tropical Salsa
1 cup finely minced fresh pineapple
1 cup finely minced fresh papaya
½ red onion, finely diced
3 cloves fresh garlic, finely minced
1 red bell pepper, finely diced
1 jalapeño chile, finely diced, do not remove seeds or ribs
2 small, firm plum tomatoes, seeds removed, finely diced
Juice of 1 lime
Juice of ½ orange
2 tablespoons finely minced fresh cilantro
4 tablespoons finely minced fresh flat-leaf parsley
½ teaspoon sea salt
Scant pinch cracked black pepper

Tempeh
3 tablespoons avocado oil
1 tablespoon erythritol
2 teaspoons soy sauce
16 ounces tempeh, cut into 2-inch slices

1 bunch bok choy, bottom removed, rinsed well, leaves left whole

Make the salsa: Combine all ingredients in a medium bowl. Set aside to allow the flavors to develop.

Make the tempeh: Place oil, erythritol and soy sauce in a skillet over medium heat. When the mixture is hot, add tempeh and cook, turning each piece until evenly browned, 7 to 8 minutes.

While the tempeh cooks, bring a pot of water with a pinch of salt to a boil. Add bok choy and cook until the stems are crisp-tender and the green part of the leaves are wilted and bright green, 3 to 4 minutes. Drain the bok choy and slice into bite-size pieces. Arrange bok choy on a platter, and place tempeh and salsa in separate bowls. To eat, top greens with tempeh and a dollop of salsa.

Variations: Mango can work in this recipe in place of the papaya. To reduce the heat in the salsa, remove the seeds and the ribs of the chile pepper.

PER SERVING: Calories 380; Protein 22.6g; Total Fat 23.2g; Saturated Fat 3.8g; Cholesterol 0mg; Carbohydrate 2/g; Dietary Fiber 8.7g; Sodium 459mg

Mustard-Scented Chickpea Salad
MAKES 3 SERVINGS

3 tablespoons extra-virgin olive oil
1 tablespoon balsamic vinegar
2 tablespoons Dijon mustard
½ teaspoon sea salt
Scant pinch cracked black pepper
4–5 scallions, finely minced
3–4 sprigs fresh basil, leaves removed and finely shredded
1½ cups cooked or canned chickpeas
3 cups baby arugula or other bitter salad greens, rinsed well

Whisk together oil, vinegar, mustard, salt, pepper, scallions and basil. Toss chickpeas and arugula with dressing until ingredients are coated. Serve at room temperature or chilled.

PER SERVING: Calories 322; Protein 11.5g; Total Fat 17.1g; Saturated Fat 2g; Cholesterol 0mg; Carbohydrate 32.8g; Dietary Fiber 6.9g; Sodium 655mg

Orange-Balsamic Glazed Tempeh over Greens
MAKES 4 SERVINGS

¼ cup frozen orange juice concentrate

¼ cup balsamic vinegar

1 tablespoon avocado oil

½ teaspoon soy sauce

2 cloves fresh garlic, crushed

1 tablespoon finely minced fresh basil

1 teaspoon finely minced fresh flat-leaf parsley

24 ounces tempeh, cut into 4 (6-ounce) slices

2 bunches kale or collards, rinsed well, stems trimmed, left whole

2 tablespoons fresh lemon juice

Combine orange juice concentrate, vinegar, oil, soy sauce, garlic, basil and parsley in a skillet over medium heat. When the mixture is hot, arrange tempeh slices in the mixture and cook until browned, about 4 minutes. Turn and brown on the other side, about 4 minutes more.

While the tempeh braises, place about ½-inch water and a pinch of salt in the bottom of a saucepan and bring to a boil. Add greens and steam until they are just wilted and bright green, about 3 minutes. Drain well and slice into bite-size pieces. Arrange greens on a platter. Arrange tempeh slices on top of greens and sprinkle with lemon juice. Serve hot.

PER SERVING: Calories 378; Protein 33.1g; Total Fat 19g; Saturated Fat 4g; Cholesterol 0mg; Carbohydrate 24.8g; Dietary Fiber 10.6g; Sodium 73mg

Baked Tofu with Moroccan Spices in Jicama and Ginger Slaw
MAKES 5 SERVINGS

Baked Tofu

8 ounces extra-firm tofu, sliced into 6 pieces

1½ tablespoons soy sauce

¼ red onion, finely minced

2 cloves fresh garlic, crushed

1 teaspoon ground cumin

1 teaspoon chili powder

1 teaspoon avocado oil

Jicama and Ginger Slaw

½ medium jicama, peeled, cut into fine julienne pieces

1 carrot, cut into fine julienne pieces

1 red bell pepper, roasted (see Note, page 153), cut into fine julienne
   pieces

1 cup finely shredded red cabbage

2 tablespoons finely minced cilantro

4 tablespoons avocado oil

2 tablespoons fresh ginger juice (see Note, below)

1 teaspoon red wine vinegar

1 teaspoon soy sauce

1 teaspoon brown rice syrup

1 tablespoon fresh lime juice

Preheat oven to 375 degrees. Lightly oil a rimmed baking sheet.

Arrange the tofu slices in a shallow baking dish. Whisk together soy sauce, red onion, garlic, cumin, chili powder and oil until ingredients are well-combined. Spoon mixture over tofu to cover. Allow to stand for 10 minutes. Drain and arrange tofu on the prepared baking sheet and bake until well-browned at the edges, about 35 minutes. Turn tofu slices and bake for another 10 minutes. Cool tofu until you can handle it and then shred it into irregular pieces, like shredded chicken.

While the tofu bakes, make the slaw: Place vegetables and cilantro in a mixing bowl. Whisk together oil, ginger juice, vinegar, soy sauce, syrup and lime juice until smooth. Toss vegetables with dressing and shredded tofu; transfer to a serving platter.

Note: To extract ginger juice, grate fresh ginger and squeeze out the juice.

PER SERVING: Calories 189; Protein 5.2g; Total Fat 14.7g; Saturated Fat 1.7g; Cholesterol 0mg; Carbohydrate 11g; Dietary Fiber 4g; Sodium 411mg

Pan-Seared Tofu with Soy-Ginger Glaze

MAKES 4 SERVINGS

Soy-Ginger Glaze
¼ cup soy sauce
¼ cup spring or filtered water
Juice and zest of 1 orange
2 tablespoons erythritol
1 teaspoon dark sesame oil
2 teaspoons fresh ginger juice

2 tablespoons avocado oil
1 pound extra-firm tofu, sliced into 8 (½-inch-thick) slices

2 to 3 scallions, thinly sliced on the diagonal

Make the glaze: Place all ingredients in a saucepan over low heat. Cook, stirring frequently, until erythritol has dissolved, about 4 minutes. Keep glaze on very low heat while preparing tofu.

Heat oil in a cast-iron skillet over medium heat. Pat tofu slices dry with a kitchen towel and lay them in the hot oil. Cook until browned, about 6 minutes. Turn and brown tofu slices on the other side, about 5 minutes. Transfer to a serving platter and spoon glaze over top. Sprinkle with scallions. Serve immediately.

Note: If you do not have a cast-iron skillet, get one. I am not a fan of nonstick skillets but you can use one for this recipe. Stainless steel skillets will cause sticking and not work so well in this recipe.

PER SERVING: Calories 186; Protein 11.1g; Total Fat 13.6g; Saturated Fat 1.8g; Cholesterol 0mg; Carbohydrate 7.5g; Dietary Fiber 1g; Sodium 923mg

Stir-Fried Tofu with Soy-Simmered Shiitakes and Wasabi Sauce

MAKES 3 SERVINGS

Soy-Simmered Shiitakes

12 dried shiitake mushrooms

2 cups spring or filtered water

1 tablespoon soy sauce

1-inch piece fresh ginger, thinly sliced

½ teaspoon dark sesame oil

Stir-Fried Tofu

1 tablespoon avocado oil

2 cloves fresh garlic, crushed

2 teaspoons fresh ginger juice (see Note, page 183)

½ red onion, cut into thin half-moon slices

Soy sauce

1 teaspoon brown rice syrup

1 small carrot, cut into fine julienne pieces

1 stalk celery, thinly sliced on the diagonal

8 ounces extra-firm tofu, cut into 1-inch cubes

2–3 scallions, thinly sliced on the diagonal

Wasabi Sauce

¼ cup spring or filtered water

½ tablespoon wasabi powder

½ tablespoon soy sauce

1 teaspoon brown rice syrup

2 teaspoons dark sesame oil

1–1½ cups cooked brown basmati rice

Make Soy-Simmered Shiitakes: Soak mushrooms in the water until soft, about 15 minutes. Add to a saucepan with soy sauce, ginger slices and sesame oil and place over medium heat. Reduce heat to low and simmer for

15 minutes. Drain and discard cooking broth. Cool enough to handle and slice thinly.

Make the tofu: Heat avocado oil over medium heat. Add garlic, ginger juice, red onion and a splash of soy sauce and sauté until the onion is translucent, about 3 minutes. Stir in syrup until well-incorporated. Stir in carrot and a splash of soy sauce and sauté for 1 minute. Stir in celery and a splash of soy sauce and sauté for 1 minute. Stir in tofu, season with 2 teaspoons soy sauce and stir-fry for 3 minutes to warm tofu through. Stir in scallions and cook until they wilt.

Make Wasabi Sauce: Whisk ingredients together until well-combined. Stir Wasabi Sauce and mushrooms into tofu. Serve immediately over a bed of rice.

PER SERVING: Calories 439; Protein 17g; Total Fat 18.8g; Saturated Fat 2.9g; Cholesterol 0mg; Carbohydrate 55.9g; Dietary Fiber 6.9g; Sodium 792mg

Pinto-Bean Chili with Fried Mushrooms

MAKES 5 SERVINGS

Pinto-Bean Chili
2 teaspoons extra-virgin olive oil
3 cloves fresh garlic, crushed
½ red onion, cut into small dice
Sea salt
1 teaspoon chili powder
1 teaspoon ground cumin
1 teaspoon dried oregano
1 small jalapeño chile, minced, seeds and spines removed
1 red bell pepper, roasted (see Note, page 153), diced
1 (15-ounce) can diced tomatoes
3 tablespoons tomato paste
1½ cups pinto beans, rinsed well, soaked for 1 hour in hot water
¼ cup quinoa, rinsed well
3–3½ cups spring or filtered water
1 bay leaf

1 teaspoon sweet paprika

2 teaspoons unsweetened cocoa powder

Fried Mushrooms

4 tablespoons avocado oil

12 fresh shiitake mushrooms, thinly sliced

Sea salt

Cracked black pepper

3 to 4 sprigs fresh flat-leaf parsley, finely minced, for garnish

Make the chili: Place oil, garlic and onion in a soup pot over medium heat. When the onion sizzles, add a pinch of salt and sauté until translucent, about 3 minutes. Add chili powder, cumin, oregano, chile, bell pepper and a pinch of salt and sauté for 1 minute. Add tomatoes and tomato paste and stir to dissolve paste. Add beans, quinoa, water, bay leaf, paprika and cocoa powder and stir well. Bring to a boil; cover and reduce heat to low. Cook until beans are creamy and soft, about 1 hour. Season with 1 teaspoon salt or less and simmer for 5 to 7 minutes more.

While the chili cooks, make the mushrooms: Heat oil in a skillet over medium heat. Add mushrooms and a pinch of salt. Cook, stirring constantly, until the mushrooms are golden brown and the edges are beginning to crisp, about 15 minutes. Season with ½ teaspoon salt or less and black pepper. Stir to distribute seasoning.

To serve the chili, spoon into individual bowls and garnish with fried mushrooms and parsley.

Note: You can substitute canned organic pinto beans in this recipe to shorten the cooking time to 30 minutes. Instead of 3 cups water, add only enough water to generously cover the ingredients to create a creamy chili.

PER SERVING: Calories 189; Protein 7.9g; Total Fat 3.13g; Saturated Fat .47g; Cholesterol 0mg; Carbohydrate 35.5g; Dietary Fiber 8.9g; Sodium 1,017mg

Barbecued Tempeh Sandwiches

MAKES 4 SERVINGS; 8 IF SERVING HALF SANDWICHES

Barbecue Sauce

⅓ cup tomato paste

2 teaspoons spring or filtered water

1 tablespoon erythritol

1 teaspoon avocado oil

1 teaspoon apple cider vinegar

1 teaspoon Dijon mustard

½ teaspoon chili powder

½ teaspoon soy sauce

2 cloves fresh garlic, very finely minced

Avocado oil

8 ounces tempeh, cut in half lengthwise and pieces cut in half to create 4 slices

1 red onion, cut into thin half-moon slices

2 red bell peppers, roasted (see Note, page 153), cut into thin ribbon slices

4 whole grain burger buns

4 leaves romaine lettuce

4 tomato slices

Prepare Barbecue Sauce: Place all ingredients in a small saucepan over low heat. Cook, stirring constantly, until erythritol dissolves, about 4 minutes. Cool slightly.

Lightly oil a cast-iron griddle and place over medium heat. Brush tempeh slices with barbecue sauce on both sides and lay on griddle. Toss onion and bell peppers with the remaining barbecue sauce and arrange on griddle to cook. Cook the tempeh until heated through and the edges are beginning to brown, 4 minutes on each side. Cook the onion and bell peppers, stirring constantly, until they are wilted and beginning to brown, 6 to 7 minutes.

Make the sandwiches: Lay burger buns open on a dry work surface. Lay a lettuce leaf and tomato slice on each bottom. Top each with a tempeh slab and spoon onion and bell peppers evenly over each sandwich. Serve immediately.

PER FULL SERVING: Calories 285; Protein 16g; Total Fat 10.9g; Saturated Fat 1.9g; Cholesterol 0mg; Carbohydrate 36.3g; Dietary Fiber 8.2g; Sodium 307mg

Nut-Crusted Tofu with Szechuan-Style Vegetables

MAKES 4 SERVINGS

1 pound extra-firm tofu

¼ cup finely chopped almonds

Pinch sea salt

2 tablespoons avocado oil

1 yellow onion, cut into thin half-moon slices

2 cloves fresh garlic, thinly sliced

1 tablespoon finely minced fresh ginger

½ teaspoon crushed red pepper flakes

1 cup thinly sliced button mushrooms

1 cup fine matchstick pieces zucchini

1 cup fine matchstick pieces fresh daikon

1 medium carrot, cut into fine matchstick pieces

2 cups small broccoli florets

2 tablespoons fruit-sweetened orange marmalade

1 tablespoon soy sauce

2 teaspoons arrowroot, dissolved in small amount cold water

Preheat oven to 275 degrees.

Slice tofu into 8 equal slices. Wrap in a kitchen towel for 5 to 10 minutes to absorb water. Mix almonds with ¼ teaspoon salt. Dredge tofu slices in ground almonds, pressing lightly so the nuts stick.

Heat 1 tablespoon of the oil in a cast-iron skillet over medium heat. When the oil is hot, lay tofu slices in hot oil and cook until browned, about 2 minutes per side. Transfer tofu to a baking sheet and place in the oven while preparing the vegetables.

Wipe out the skillet, add remaining oil and place over medium heat. Add onion, garlic, ginger, red pepper flakes and a pinch of salt and sauté until the onion is translucent, about 3 minutes. Stir in mushrooms and a pinch of salt and sauté for 2 minutes. Stir in zucchini and a pinch of salt and sauté for 1 minute. Stir in daikon and a pinch of salt and sauté for 1 minute. Stir in carrot and a pinch of salt and sauté for 1 minute. Stir in broccoli and a pinch of salt and sauté until bright green, 2 to 3 minutes (depending on size of florets). Whisk together marmalade, soy sauce and arrowroot. Stir mixture into vegetables and cook, stirring, until the sauce is clear and coats the vegetables with a thin glaze, about 2 minutes.

Spoon vegetables onto a shallow platter and top with tofu slices.

PER SERVING: Calories 255; Protein 14.6g; Total Fat 17.2g; Saturated Fat 1.9g; Cholesterol 0mg; Carbohydrate 20.2g; Dietary Fiber 4.6g; Sodium 473mg

Fresh Fava Bean, Onion and Fennel Saute

MAKES 4 SERVINGS

2 teaspoons extra-virgin olive oil

2 cloves fresh garlic, crushed

1 red onion, cut into thin half-moon slices

1 yellow onion, cut into thin half-moon slices

Sea salt

Grated zest of 1 lemon

¼ cup dry white wine

1 medium fennel bulb, stems removed, 2 tablespoons of fronds reserved
    and bulb thinly sliced

1 cup shelled fresh fava beans

2 teaspoons fresh lemon juice (optional)

Place oil, garlic and onions in a deep skillet over medium heat. When the onions begin to sizzle, add a pinch of salt and sauté until onions are translucent, about 5 minutes. Stir in lemon zest and wine. Add fennel and a pinch of salt and sauté for 1 minute. Cover; reduce heat to low and simmer for 5 minutes. Stir in fava beans and ⅔ teaspoon salt. Cook, stirring, until fava beans are tender, 3 to 4 minutes. Remove from heat and stir in reserved fennel fronds. Spoon vegetables into a serving bowl and sprinkle with lemon juice (if using).

PER SERVING: Calories 83; Protein 2.7g; Total Fat 2.7g; Saturated Fat 0g; Cholesterol 0mg; Carbohydrate 10.8g; Dietary Fiber 3.64g; Sodium 495mg

Tofu, Asparagus and Red Pepper Stir-Fry over Quinoa

MAKES 4 SERVINGS

Quinoa

1 cup quinoa, rinsed very well (see Note, page 157)

2 cups spring or filtered water

Pinch sea salt

2 teaspoons chia seeds (optional) (see Note, page 158)

Tofu, Asparagus and Red Pepper Stir-Fry

1 tablespoon avocado oil

3 cloves fresh garlic, thinly sliced

3 tablespoons fresh ginger, cut into fine matchstick pieces

1 red onion, cut into thin half-moon slices

Soy sauce

2 red bell peppers, roasted (see Note, page 153), cut into thin ribbon slices

1 pound extra-firm tofu, cut into 1-inch cubes

8–10 stalks asparagus, tips snapped off, stalks thinly sliced diagonally

Grated zest of 1 orange

2 tablespoons fresh lemon juice

Make quinoa: Place quinoa and water in a saucepan and bring to a boil. Add salt, cover and reduce heat to low. Cook until all the water has been absorbed and quinoa has opened (little tails will form that look like tadpoles), about 20 minutes. Remove from heat and stir in chia seeds (if using).

Make stir-fry while the quinoa cooks: Heat oil in a deep skillet or wok over medium heat. Add garlic, ginger, onion and a splash of soy sauce and sauté until the onion is translucent, about 3 minutes. Stir in bell peppers, a splash of soy sauce and sauté for 1 minute.

Add tofu but do not stir in; season with 1 teaspoon soy sauce. Cover; reduce heat to low and simmer until tofu is cooked through, about 7 minutes. Add asparagus, orange zest and soy sauce to your taste (but do not make it salty). Cover and cook until asparagus is bright green, about 4 minutes. Remove from heat and gently stir in lemon juice, taking care not to break tofu.

To serve, arrange quinoa in a shallow platter and spoon the stir-fry over top.

PER SERVING: Calories 325; Protein 16.7g; Total Fat 11.6g; Saturated Fat 1.5g; Cholesterol 0mg; Carbohydrate 42.2g; Dietary Fiber 5.8g; Sodium 150mg

Black Bean Burritos
MAKES 6 SERVINGS

1 tablespoon extra-virgin olive oil

2 cloves fresh garlic, finely minced

1 red onion, cut into thin half-moon slices

Sea salt

1 cup minced cremini mushrooms

1 cup minced portobello mushrooms, gills removed

1 tablespoon chili powder

1 cup canned diced tomatoes

1 small jalapeño chile, seeds and ribs removed, minced

1 red bell pepper, roasted (see Note, page 153), cut into small dice

1½ cups cooked or canned black turtle beans

4–5 sprigs fresh cilantro, finely minced

6 whole grain, low-fat soft tortillas or wraps, warmed in the oven

6 tablespoons grated vegan Monterey Jack cheese alternative

Place oil, garlic and onion in a deep skillet over medium heat. When the onion begins to sizzle, add a pinch of salt and sauté until translucent, about 3 minutes. Stir in mushrooms, chili powder and a pinch of salt and sauté until the mushrooms release their moisture and begin to wilt, about 3 minutes. Stir in tomatoes, jalapeño chile, bell pepper and a pinch of salt. Add beans, cover and reduce heat to low. Simmer for 10 to 12 minutes. Season with 1 teaspoon salt and simmer, stirring often, for 3 minutes more. Remove from heat and stir in cilantro.

To serve, lay tortillas on individual plates and mound bean mixture evenly down the center of each. Sprinkle 1 tablespoon cheese alternative on each burrito. Fold the short ends of the tortillas over filling and roll the tortilla, jelly-roll style, to enclose the filling.

PER SERVING: Calories 222; Protein 8.7g; Total Fat 5.5g; Saturated Fat .65g; Cholesterol 0mg; Carbohydrate 40.4g; Dietary Fiber 6.2g; Sodium 1,112mg

Lentils with Greens
MAKES 4 TO 5 SERVINGS

2 teaspoons extra-virgin olive oil

2 cloves fresh garlic, crushed

1 red onion, cut into small dice

Sea salt

2 stalks celery, cut into small dice

1 medium carrot, cut into small dice

1 red bell pepper, roasted (see Note, page 153), cut into small dice

1 cup green or brown lentils, rinsed well

3 cups spring or filtered water

1 bay leaf

1 small bunch escarole, rinsed very well, hand-shredded into bite-size
   pieces

Place oil, garlic and onion in a deep skillet over medium heat. When the onion begins to sizzle, add a pinch of salt and sauté until translucent, about 3 minutes. Stir in celery and a pinch of salt and sauté for 1 minute. Stir in carrot and a pinch of salt and sauté for 1 minute. Stir in bell pepper and a pinch of salt and sauté for 1 minute. Add lentils, water and bay leaf and bring to a boil. Cover and reduce heat to low. Cook until lentils are soft and all the water has been absorbed, about 45 minutes. Season with 1 teaspoon salt; stir in escarole and cook, covered, until escarole is tender and wilted, about 4 minutes. Stir well to combine and transfer to a serving bowl.

PER SERVING: Calories 218; Protein 14.8g; Total Fat 3g; Saturated Fat .43g; Cholesterol 0mg; Carbohydrate 35.3g; Dietary Fiber 17.3g; Sodium 754mg

White Beans in Spicy Tomato Sauce
MAKES 3 SERVINGS

2 teaspoons extra-virgin olive oil

4 cloves fresh garlic, crushed

½ red onion, cut into small dice

Sea salt

Generous pinch crushed red pepper flakes

2 tablespoons dry white wine

1 cup canned diced tomatoes

2 cups cooked or canned cannellini beans

4 sprigs fresh oregano, leaves removed, left whole

Place oil, garlic and onion in a saucepan over medium heat. When the onion begins to sizzle, add a pinch of salt and sauté until translucent, about 3 minutes. Add red pepper flakes and white wine and cook, stirring, until wine reduces to a syrup, about 3 minutes. Add tomatoes and beans and bring to a boil. Reduce heat and cook just until the beans become creamy, 15 to 20 minutes. Add 1 teaspoon salt and cook, stirring gently, for 3 to 5 minutes. Stir in oregano and transfer to a serving bowl.

PER SERVING: Calories 230; Protein 12.7g; Total Fat 3.6g; Saturated Fat .55g; Cholesterol 0mg; Carbohydrate 36.9g; Dietary Fiber 9.3g; Sodium 928mg

Fried Tempeh over Cold Sesame Noodles
MAKES 4 SERVINGS

Sesame Sauce

6 scallions, finely minced

2 tablespoons soy sauce

1 teaspoon hot pepper sauce

1 tablespoon sesame tahini

1 tablespoon sesame oil

1 tablespoon brown rice vinegar

1 teaspoon brown rice syrup
Spring or filtered water

Fried Tempeh
4 tablespoons avocado oil
1 teaspoon soy sauce
1 teaspoon brown rice syrup
8 ounces tempeh, cut into 1-inch cubes

8 ounces whole wheat udon noodles, cooked al dente, rinsed well after cooking
3–4 sprigs flat-leaf parsley, coarsely chopped, for garnish

Make the sauce: Whisk together all ingredients in a small bowl, slowly adding water to thin the sauce to a creamy consistency. Set aside.

Make the tempeh: Heat oil, soy sauce and syrup in a skillet over medium heat. Add tempeh and cook, turning, until the tempeh browns on all sides, about 5 minutes.

Toss noodles with sauce and tempeh. Serve garnished with parsley.

PER SERVING: Calories 304; Protein 12g; Total Fat 25.6g; Saturated Fat 3.7g; Cholesterol 0mg; Carbohydrate 10.9g; Dietary Fiber 3.8g; Sodium 574mg

Edamame Hummus
MAKES 4 SERVINGS

2 cups shelled edamame
1½ tablespoons sesame tahini
2 teaspoons fresh ginger juice (see Note, page 183)
1 tablespoon plus 1 teaspoon extra-virgin olive oil
1 clove fresh garlic, crushed
½ teaspoon sea salt
Generous pinch cracked black pepper
1 tablespoon fresh lemon juice
2 tablespoons finely minced fresh flat-leaf parsley
Belgian endive leaves, cucumber slices, carrot and celery sticks or pita
    points, to serve

Bring a pot of water to a boil with a pinch of salt. Add edamame and boil for 5 minutes. Drain well and cool to room temperature.

In a food processor, combine cooked edamame, tahini, ginger juice, 1 tablespoon oil, garlic, salt, pepper and lemon juice and puree until smooth. Transfer to a small bowl and fold in parsley.

To serve hummus, mound in the center of a platter and drizzle remaining 1 teaspoon oil over top. Surround with vegetables or pita points.

PER SERVING: Calories 266; Protein 17.2g; Total Fat 16g; Saturated Fat .82g; Cholesterol 0mg; Carbohydrate 15.1g; Dietary Fiber 6g; Sodium 390mg

Curried Tofu Spring Rolls with Pineapple Sauce
MAKES 8 SERVINGS

8 ounces extra-firm tofu, cut into thin strips

3 scallions, diced

1 tablespoon finely minced ginger

3 cloves fresh garlic, crushed

1 teaspoon brown rice syrup

1 tablespoon soy sauce

Generous pinch saffron

3 tablespoons red curry paste

1 teaspoon avocado oil

1 cup green beans, ends trimmed, split lengthwise

1 medium carrot, cut into fine matchstick pieces

Pineapple Sauce

½ cup unsweetened pineapple juice

4 tablespoons arrowroot

¼ cup erythritol

1 teaspoon avocado oil

2 tablespoons red wine vinegar

4 sheets thawed phyllo dough, each cut into 4 equal squares
Avocado oil, for brushing
1 cup mung bean sprouts

Arrange tofu in a baking dish. Whisk together scallions, ginger, garlic, syrup, soy sauce, saffron, curry paste and oil. Spoon over tofu and toss gently to coat. Set aside to marinate for 10 minutes.

While the tofu marinates, bring a pot of water to a boil with a pinch of salt. Add green beans and boil until bright green, about 2 minutes. Remove beans, drain and set aside. Add carrot to pot and boil for 2 minutes. Drain and mix with beans.

Transfer tofu and marinade to a skillet, and place over medium heat. Cook, stirring, for 5 minutes to flavor tofu. Transfer to a serving plate to cool to room temperature.

Make the sauce: Combine juice, arrowroot, erythritol and oil in a saucepan over low heat. Cook, whisking constantly, until the erythritol dissolves and the mixture thickens, about 3 minutes. Remove from heat and whisk in vinegar. Cover and set aside to cool. (You must cover it so a skin doesn't form on the sauce.)

Preheat oven to 375 degrees and line a baking sheet with unbleached parchment paper.

Lay 1 square of phyllo on a dry work surface. Brush lightly with oil and lay another phyllo square on top. Arrange green beans and carrots diagonally in the center; mound tofu on top and lay mung bean sprouts on top of the tofu. Fold short corners over filling and roll, jelly-roll style to wrap phyllo around filling. Lay on baking sheet, seam side down. Repeat with the rest of the phyllo and filling to create 8 spring rolls. Arrange on baking sheet; avoid having the rolls touch. Lightly brush with oil and bake until pastry is golden and crispy, 15 to 20 minutes. Remove from oven and serve with Pineapple Sauce on the side.

PER SERVING: Calories 116; Protein 3.9g; Total Fat 2.7g; Saturated Fat .4g; Cholesterol 0mg; Carbohydrate 16.8g; Dietary Fiber 1.8g; Sodium 380mg

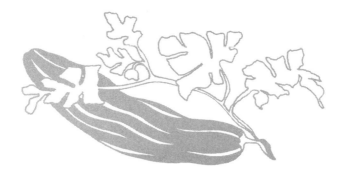

VITALITY THROUGH VEGGIES

If you want to really change your life, your body, your health and your think-ing; if you really want to rethink every single thing you know about disease prevention, weight management, aging well, fitness and living green, then this is the section for you. Of all the changes you can make in your life, eat-ing vegetables will yield the most dramatic effects.

Not only delicious and a fine and elegant way to feed yourself, vegeta-bles also aid us in all aspects of our lives. Whether you are an athlete who stresses the body, a couch potato who stresses about being fat, a stressed-out parent, a stressed-out student, a stressed-out executive, a stressed-out doctor or nurse or teacher or...you get the idea. Regardless of your current lifestyle or emotional state, eating vegetables—lots of them—on a regular basis will change you completely.

People who eat a lot of vegetables have greater antioxidant status, which better equips them to deal with the damage caused by life stress (and exer-cise stress). Oxidative reactions that occur with stress produce free radicals. These are volatile molecules that damage cells and DNA causing degenera-tion of tissue, which leads to premature aging, weakness and disease.

When you eat vegetables, variety is the key to achieving and main-taining your youthful vitality. Our generous planet has provided us with so much to choose from, and each vegetable brings unique nutrients and energy to your body; enjoy the bounty! In this section, I have broken the vegetables into three parts; root vegetables, ground vegetables and leafy vegetables. You can mix and match within your plan and still get all the variety you need to be strong and vital.

Cooking Veggies

There are some basic techniques that will ensure that your veggies are cooked to perfection every time, but don't stress. We're not splitting the atom; we're just cooking. With these basic techniques at your fingertips, you will master the kitchen and these recipes in no time flat.

STEAMING

Steaming is a very simple and efficient method for cooking greens without any fuss and with no added fat and calories. It also preserves nutrients and flavor and cooks vegetables to light, tender perfection.

Bring a small amount of water to a rolling boil with a pinch of salt. In a metal steamer or using a bamboo steamer, cook the vegetables above the water until just wilted and tender, with bright color still retained. This method of cooking is best for more delicate vegetables like dark leafy greens, broccoli, cauliflower, snow peas and snap peas. Harder vegetables can be steamed if they are first cut into thin, delicate pieces. You are limited only by what you can imagine.

BOILING

Boiling vegetables involves submerging them entirely in boiling water and cooking until they are at the tenderness you desire. Boiling is a light way to cook vegetables and is especially nice for breakfast because the resulting vegetables are tender, moist and easy to digest.

Bring a pot of water to a boil with a pinch of salt (to keep the flavor and nutrients in the vegetables). Cook vegetables until just tender, usually 3 to 5 minutes, depending on the vegetable, how hard it is and how it is cut. For example, medium cauliflower and broccoli florets will cook to perfection in 4 to 5 minutes. Dark leafy greens will cook in 2 to 3 minutes. With greens like kale and collards, remember to boil them whole so that they retain more of their nutrients. (Once you cut them, they begin to lose their strength.) Cut them after cooking for the best results. Harder vegetables like medium-size chopped chunks of carrots, rutabaga and other roots can take as long as 5 minutes; if they are cut in bigger pieces, they will take even longer.

BLANCHING

Blanching is the quickest of all cooking methods and used only to just wilt delicate vegetables or vegetables that are delicately cut. If I want to wilt watercress, a simple dip into boiling, salted water will do the trick. When I want to take the bite out of red onion slices for a salad or when I am freezing fresh herbs, I dip these delicate vegetables in boiling salted water. This is the method to use when you do not want to cook a vegetable too much or when the vegetable is so delicate that cooking will quickly turn it to mush.

SAUTÉING

Sauté means "to jump" in French. This lively form of cooking requires a bit of oil and a very hot pan. In this cooking method you sear the vegetable, sealing nutrients and flavor in, but also imparting the richness of oil without the calories of frying. This is a great way to get the satisfaction you want without adding a lot of fat to a recipe.

OVEN ROASTING

One of the most satisfying ways to cook vegetables, oven roasting forces the natural sugars in vegetables to the surface and creates a deeply sweet and satisfying result. Most vegetables yield the best results when roasted at 350 F (180 C) for 1 to 1½ hours.

GRILLING

A hot pan, stovetop griddle or outdoor grill sears the vegetables, sealing in flavor and nutrients and giving them a smoky, satisfying flavor without adding a ton of calories.

FRYING

An occasional cooking method at best, frying results in richly flavored vegetables that are hard to beat, but the calories can really add up, so use this cooking method sparingly. A healthy oil, like avocado, is brought to a high temperature (at least 315 F (160 C)) and the food is fried until crispy. I find that slowly bringing the oil to temperature is the most effective way of getting your oil truly hot. This is an important step, because if the oil is very hot the vegetables will cook quickly and not absorb a ton of oil and calories.

Radical Roots

Root vegetables drill deep into the soil, drawing minerals and vitamins from the earth into their cores. They provide us not only with nutrients and fiber, but with a grounded, strengthening energy that can't be beat. In Chinese medicine, these vegetables are said to nourish the function of the digestive tract, reproductive system, muscles and bones, so you can be strong.

Roasted Carrots, Parsnips and Onions

MAKES 5 TO 6 SERVINGS

2 medium carrots, cut into 1-inch irregular chunks

2 medium parsnips, cut into 1-inch irregular chunks

2 red onions, cut lengthwise into 8 wedges

8 cloves fresh garlic, peeled, left whole

2 tablespoons extra-virgin olive oil

1 tablespoon balsamic vinegar

1 teaspoon sea salt

1 teaspoon fresh lemon juice

3 to 4 sprigs fresh flat-leaf parsley, coarsely minced, for garnish

Preheat oven to 375 degrees.

Place vegetables in a mixing bowl and add oil, vinegar and salt. Toss to coat. Arrange vegetables in a shallow baking dish, avoiding overlap. Cover tightly and bake for 45 minutes. Remove cover and return vegetables to the oven for 10 to 15 minutes to brown the edges lightly. Remove from oven and toss gently with lemon juice and parsley. Serve immediately.

Note: Leftover roasted vegetables make a nice base for a soup or stew.

PER SERVING: Calories 107; Protein 1.4g; Total Fat 5.8g; Saturated Fat .8g; Cholesterol 0mg; Carbohydrate 13.2g; Dietary Fiber 2.9g; Sodium 474mg

Skinny Sweet Potato Fries

MAKES 6 SERVINGS

5 medium sweet potatoes, rinsed, cut into ½-inch-thick spears

2 tablespoons extra-virgin olive oil

½ teaspoon sea salt

Preheat oven to 425 degrees. Line a shallow baking sheet with foil and lightly oil it.

Toss sweet potato pieces with oil and salt and arrange on baking sheet, avoiding overlap. Bake for 30 minutes, turning once to ensure even browning. Serve hot.

Variations: You can toss ½ teaspoon dried basil, oregano or other favorite herbs with the sweet potato mixture. For spicy fries, add ½ teaspoon chili powder. The spice actually enhances the sweet flavor of the sweet potatoes.

PER SERVING: Calories 156; Protein 1.8g; Total Fat 5g; Saturated Fat 1g; Cholesterol 0mg; Carbohydrate 26.3g; Dietary Fiber 3.2g; Sodium 206mg

Mashed Sweet Potatoes with Orange
MAKES 4 TO 5 SERVINGS

2 pounds unpeeled sweet potatoes, rinsed well

1 tablespoon brown rice syrup

1 tablespoon avocado oil

½ teaspoon sea salt

Generous pinch cracked black pepper

2 tablespoons fresh orange juice

½ orange, peeled, thinly sliced into half-moon pieces, for garnish

Place a metal steamer basket in the bottom of a pot with enough water to almost reach the bottom of the basket. Cut sweet potatoes into chunks and steam until tender. Drain well and peel chunks when cool enough to handle. Combine sweet potatoes with remaining ingredients in a bowl and mash or beat until well blended and creamy. Serve hot, garnished with orange slices.

PER SERVING: Calories 292; Protein 3.9g; Total Fat 4.2g; Saturated Fat .56g; Cholesterol 0mg; Carbohydrate 60.6g; Dietary Fiber 7.2g; Sodium 317mg

Jicama Slaw with Mustard-Fennel Vinaigrette

MAKES 4 TO 5 SERVINGS

1 cup julienne jicama (see Note, below)

1 cup shredded radicchio

1 large carrot, cut into very fine julienne

1 cup finely shredded green cabbage

2 Belgian endive, shredded

4–5 scallions, thinly sliced on the diagonal

3–4 sprigs basil, leaves removed and shredded

3–4 sprigs fresh flat-leaf parsley, coarsely chopped

Mustard-Fennel Vinaigrette

1 teaspoon fennel seed

1 tablespoon red wine vinegar

1 tablespoon balsamic vinegar

1 tablespoon fresh lemon juice

1 tablespoon Dijon mustard

1 clove fresh garlic, very finely minced

6 tablespoons extra-virgin olive oil

½ teaspoon sea salt, or to taste

Generous pinch cracked black pepper

Mix vegetables and herbs together in a large bowl and set aside.

Prepare the vinaigrette: Pan-toast fennel seed in a dry skillet over medium heat until fragrant, about 5 minutes. Transfer to a mortar and pestle bowl or spice grinder and grind into a fine powder. Whisk fennel with remaining ingredients in a small bowl. Add vinaigrette to vegetable mixture and toss to coat. Serve at room temperature or chilled.

Note: Jicama is also known as Mexican potato and can be found in most produce sections. Though it looks like a large potato with pale brown skin, it does not need to be peeled, but you can. If you cannot find jicama, you can substitute fresh daikon in its place.

PER SERVING: Calories 237; Protein 1.7g; Total Fat 21.6g; Saturated Fat 2.99g; Cholesterol 0mg; Carbohydrate 10.3g; Dietary Fiber 3.8g; Sodium 406mg

Baked Carrots and Butternut Squash with Cinnamon-Chili Oil

MAKES 5 TO 6 SERVINGS

Cinnamon-Chili Oil

5 tablespoons avocado oil

1 tablespoon brown rice syrup

3 fresh garlic cloves, finely minced

1 teaspoon chili powder

½ teaspoon ground cinnamon

½ teaspoon sea salt

2 medium carrots, cut into 1-inch irregular chunks

2 cups 1-inch cubes unpeeled butternut squash

1 yellow onion, cut into 12 wedges

Preheat oven to 375 degrees.

Make Cinnamon-Chili Oil: Place all ingredients in a small saucepan over medium heat and cook, whisking frequently, for 5 minutes.

Toss oil with vegetables in a mixing bowl and spoon into a shallow baking dish, avoiding overlap. Cover tightly and bake for 45 minutes. Remove cover and return to oven for about 15 minutes to lightly brown. Serve hot.

PER SERVING: Calories 184; Protein 1.2g; Total Fat 14.2g; Saturated Fat 1.7g; Cholesterol 0mg; Carbohydrate 11.9g; Dietary Fiber 3.4g; Sodium 247mg

Daikon, Carrot and Winter Squash Stew

MAKES 4 TO 5 SERVINGS

1-inch piece of kombu or 1 bay leaf

1 dried shiitake mushroom, soaked until tender, stem removed, left whole

1 cup 1-inch chunks fresh daikon

1 large carrot, cut into 1-inch irregular chunks

2 cups 1-inch cubes unpeeled winter squash (butternut, Hokkaido, buttercup or delicate)

Spring or filtered water

2 teaspoons soy sauce

1 teaspoon fresh lemon juice

3–4 sprigs fresh flat-leaf parsley, coarsely chopped

Place kombu in a heavy pot. Layer vegetables over kombu in the order listed. Add enough water to just cover the bottom of the pot (do not exceed ⅛ inch in the pot) and a splash of soy sauce; cover and bring to a boil over medium heat. Reduce heat to low and cook until vegetables are tender, 25 to 30 minutes. Season with soy sauce; cook, uncovered, until any remaining liquid evaporates, 5 to 7 minutes more. Remove from heat and gently stir in lemon juice and parsley, taking care not to break the vegetables.

PER SERVING: Calories 49; Protein 1.4g; Total Fat .15g; Saturated Fat 0g; Cholesterol 0mg; Carbohydrate 12g; Dietary Fiber 3.5g; Sodium 168mg

Braised Carrots and Tops
MAKES 4 TO 5 SERVINGS

3 tablespoons extra-virgin olive oil

2 tablespoons balsamic vinegar

1 teaspoon sea salt

3 large carrots with tops, tops removed, hard stems removed and coarsely chopped; carrots cut into ½-inch irregular chunks

2 tablespoons fresh lemon juice

Place oil, vinegar and salt in a skillet over medium heat. Stir to combine ingredients. Arrange carrots in the skillet. Cover and listen for a strong sizzle. Reduce heat to low and cook carrots until just tender, 15 to 20 minutes.

Stir in carrot tops, cover and cook until bright green and tender, about 5 minutes. Add lemon juice and stir well to combine. Serve hot.

PER SERVING (without tops): Calories 127; Protein .69g; Total Fat 10.6g; Saturated Fat 1.5g; Cholesterol 0mg; Carbohydrate 8g; Dietary Fiber 1.86g; Sodium 598mg

Grounded!

Want to bust stress? This is the neighborhood in the plant kingdom where that happens. These mild-mannered vegetables grow close to the surface of the earth with a calm, serene energy. With comforting round shapes and delicate vines and leaves, they give you the kind of centered calm that you need to face life's little adventures. Said in Chinese medicine to nourish the function of your middle organs: spleen, pancreas, liver, lungs and stomach, these veggies will be at the core of your sanity.

Sauteed Brussels Sprout Leaves

MAKES 3 TO 4 SERVINGS

2 teaspoons extra-virgin olive oil
2 cloves fresh garlic, cut into julienne or matchstick pieces
2 shallots, cut into very thin half-moon slices
1 teaspoon sea salt
Grated zest of 1 lemon
2 red bell peppers, roasted (see Note, page 153), cut into very thin julienne or matchstick pieces
10–12 Brussels sprouts, tips trimmed, most leaves removed, cores shredded
Generous pinch cracked black pepper
2 teaspoons fresh lemon juice

Place oil, garlic and shallots in a skillet over medium heat. When the shallots begin to sizzle, add a pinch of the salt and lemon zest and sauté until translucent, about 3 minutes. Stir in bell pepper and a pinch of the salt and sauté for 1 minute. Stir in Brussels sprout leaves and cores; cover and reduce heat to low. Cook for 5 minutes. Remove cover and season with remaining salt and black pepper. Cook, stirring, for 3 minutes for flavors to develop. Remove from heat and stir in lemon juice. Serve immediately.

PER SERVING: Calories 86; Protein 3.2g; Total Fat 3.5g; Saturated Fat .5g; Cholesterol 0mg; Carbohydrate 13g; Dietary Fiber 4.3g; Sodium 785mg

Cauliflower with Cumin-Scented Oil

MAKES 5 TO 6 SERVINGS; ½ CUP OIL

Cumin-Scented Oil
½ cup avocado oil
Grated zest of 1 lemon
1 teaspoon cumin seed
½ teaspoon crushed red pepper flakes
½ teaspoon sea salt

1 head cauliflower, broken into medium florets
3 to 4 sprigs basil, leaves removes, shredded

Prepare oil: Place all ingredients in a saucepan over low heat and cook, uncovered, for 10 to 12 minutes. Turn off heat and let stand, undisturbed, for 1 hour to allow flavors to develop. Strain oil and reserve ¼ cup. Transfer remaining oil to a glass jar. Seal the jar tightly after the oil has cooled. Refrigerate leftover oil for another use. Use within 5 days.

While the oil steeps, bring a pot of water to a boil with a pinch of salt. Add cauliflower and cook until crisp-tender, about 4 minutes. Drain well and transfer to a mixing bowl. Allow to cool slightly before proceeding.

Toss cauliflower with basil and reserved ¼ cup oil.

PER SERVING: Calories 131; Protein 2.5g; Total Fat 11.5g; Saturated Fat 1.3g; Cholesterol 0mg; Carbohydrate 6.6g; Dietary Fiber 3.1g; Sodium 152mg

Artichoke Hearts with Garlic, Olive Oil and Basil

MAKES 5 TO 6 SERVINGS

2 teaspoons extra-virgin olive oil

4 cloves fresh garlic, crushed

1 red onion, cut into thin half-moon slices

Sea salt

10–12 canned artichoke hearts (in water, not oil), halved

1 cup canned diced tomatoes

Generous pinch cracked black pepper

5–7 sprigs fresh basil, leaves removed, left whole

Place oil, garlic and red onion in a deep skillet over medium heat. When the onion begins to sizzle, add a pinch of salt and sauté until translucent, about 3 minutes. Add artichoke hearts, tomatoes and black pepper. Bring to a boil; cover and reduce heat to low. Cook for 15 minutes. Season with ⅔ teaspoon salt and simmer, uncovered, for 5 minutes, stirring frequently to thicken tomatoes slightly. Stir in basil leaves and transfer to a serving bowl.

PER SERVING: Calories 54; Protein 1.8g; Total Fat 1.9g; Saturated Fat .27g; Cholesterol 0mg; Carbohydrate 8.1g; Dietary Fiber 2.3g; Sodium 566mg

Asparagus Bundles

MAKES 4 SERVINGS

1 pound asparagus, tough ends snapped off

2 long leaves from 1 small leek

Lemon Vinaigrette

1 tablespoon extra-virgin olive oil

1 tablespoon balsamic vinegar

1 teaspoon brown rice syrup

1 tablespoon fresh lemon juice

1 clove fresh garlic, very finely minced
1 small shallot, very finely minced
¼ teaspoon sea salt
Generous pinch cracked black pepper

1 red bell pepper, roasted (see Note, page 153), cut into thin ribbons
2 tablespoons coarsely chopped walnuts

Place asparagus in a skillet with water to cover and bring to a boil. Reduce heat to low and cook, covered, until bright green and crisp-tender, about 6 minutes.

While the asparagus cooks, split the leek leaves in half lengthwise and steam until wilted, about 4 minutes. Drain and cool asparagus just until you can handle it. When the asparagus is cool enough to handle, divide into 4 equal bunches. Tie a steamed leek strip around each bundle and arrange on a platter.

Prepare vinaigrette: Whisk together all ingredients and spoon over asparagus bundles.

Sprinkle with bell pepper and walnuts. Serve at room temperature.

PER SERVING: Calories 70; Protein .98g; Total Fat 6g; Saturated Fat .73g; Cholesterol 0mg; Carbohydrate 4g; Dietary Fiber .89g; Sodium 146mg

Artichokes Stuffed with Gremolata
MAKES 2 SERVINGS

Gremolata
8 tablespoons finely chopped fresh flat-leaf parsley
4 cloves fresh garlic, finely minced
4 teaspoons finely grated lemon zest
½ teaspoon sea salt

2 large globe artichokes
Spring or filtered water
1 tablespoon extra-virgin olive oil
Pinch sea salt

Prepare gremolata: Combine all ingredients in a small bowl. Mix very well. Set aside.

Cut the stems off the artichokes, flush with the bottoms, so the artichokes can stand upright. Using sharp kitchen scissors, cut the very tip off each leaf of the artichokes, up to the top quarter. Using a sharp knife, slice the top quarters off the artichokes, creating a flat top. Using a grapefruit spoon or your fingers, push open the center of the artichokes and scoop out the hairy choke.

Stuff both artichokes with equal amounts of gremolata, pushing the stuffing into as many of the crevices of the artichoke leaves as you can, pushing the remaining stuffing into the center.

Stand artichokes in a pan that is deep enough to cover them. Add water to half cover and drizzle with oil and salt. Cover and bring to a boil. Reduce heat to low and cook until artichoke leaves pull off easily, about 1 hour. Serve hot.

PER SERVING: Calories 94; Protein 6.1g; Total Fat .4g; Saturated Fat 0g; Cholesterol 0mg; Carbohydrate 20.9g; Dietary Fiber 9.79g; Sodium 806mg

Spiced Onion Marmalade
MAKES ABOUT 4 CUPS; 16 (1/4-CUP) SERVINGS

2 tablespoons extra-virgin olive oil

8–10 medium yellow onions, cut into thin half-moon slices

2 teaspoons sea salt

1 teaspoon ground cinnamon

½ teaspoon ground nutmeg

2 bay leaves

½ cup unsweetened apple juice

Place oil and onions in a large Dutch oven over low heat. When the onions begin to sizzle, add a generous pinch of the salt and cook onions, stirring until they begin to wilt, about 15 minutes. Stir in remaining salt, spices, bay leaves and apple juice. Turn heat to medium and cook, stirring frequently, until the onions are a light caramel color and are quite reduced in volume, about 2 hours. Once cooked, serve as you like. Cool the rest and store in the refrigerator. It will keep for about 2 weeks.

PER SERVING: Calories 41; Protein .65g; Total Fat 1.8g; Saturated Fat .26g; Cholesterol 0mg; Carbohydrate 5.8g; Dietary Fiber 1.1g; Sodium 290mg

Artichoke Stew with Peas
MAKES 5 SERVINGS

2 teaspoons extra-virgin olive oil
2 cloves fresh garlic, thinly sliced
1 small leek, split lengthwise, cut into 1-inch pieces, rinsed free of dirt
Sea salt
Generous pinch crushed red pepper flakes
Generous pinch crushed saffron
2 stalks celery, cut into thin oblong slices
1 medium carrot, cut into thin oblong slices
2 cups halved canned artichoke hearts (in water, not oil)
1 cup canned diced tomatoes
¼ cup spring or filtered water
4–5 sprigs fresh basil, leaves removed, left whole
1 cup fresh or frozen peas

Place oil, garlic and leek in a heavy saucepan over medium heat. When the leek begins to sizzle, add a pinch of salt, red pepper flakes and saffron and sauté until leek is quite limp, about 2 minutes. Stir in celery and a pinch of salt and sauté for 1 minute. Stir in carrot and a pinch of salt and sauté for 1 minute. Stir in artichoke hearts and tomatoes and add water. Bring to a boil. Cover; reduce heat to low and cook until carrots are tender, 12 to 15 minutes. Add ⅔ teaspoon salt and cook for 5 minutes more. Stir in basil leaves and peas and cook for 1 minute. Transfer to a serving bowl and serve hot.

PER SERVING: Calories 102; Protein 4.6g; Total Fat 2g; Saturated Fat .29g; Cholesterol 0mg; Carbohydrate 16.7g; Dietary Fiber 3.5g; Sodium 700mg

Cauliflower in Spiced Tomato Sauce

MAKES 7 TO 8 SERVINGS

Spiced Tomato Sauce
2 teaspoons extra-virgin olive oil
2 cloves fresh garlic, crushed
½ red onion, small dice
Sea salt
½ teaspoon curry powder
Generous pinch crushed saffron
2 cups canned diced tomatoes
3 tablespoons capers, drained, do not rinse
8 pitted, oil-cured black olives, coarsely chopped
3–4 sprigs fresh flat-leaf parsley, coarsely chopped

Spring or filtered water
1 medium head cauliflower, leaves trimmed, core removed, left whole

Prepare the sauce: Place oil, garlic and onion in a saucepan over medium heat. When the onion begins to sizzle, add a pinch of salt, curry powder and saffron and sauté until the onion is translucent, about 3 minutes. Stir in tomatoes, capers and olives, season with about ½ teaspoon salt and bring to a boil. Cover and reduce heat to low. Cook for 15 to 20 minutes. Remove from heat and stir in parsley.

While the sauce cooks, bring about ⅔ inch of water to a boil with a pinch of salt in a large pot. Add cauliflower and steam until you can easily pierce it with a fork, about 12 to 15 minutes (depending on the size).

Transfer cauliflower to a serving platter. Spoon sauce liberally over top and serve with the remaining sauce on the side.

PER SERVING: Calories 39; Protein .82g; Total Fat 2.1g; Saturated Fat .2g; Cholesterol 0mg; Carbohydrate 4.9g; Dietary Fiber 1.5g; Sodium 436mg

Roasted Winter Squash with Basil

MAKES 5 TO 6 SERVINGS

3 cups ½-inch cubes winter squash (Hokkaido, butternut, buttercup,
   delicata)

1 yellow onion, cut into ½-inch dice

2 teaspoons avocado oil

2 teaspoons soy sauce

Grated zest of 1 orange

1 teaspoon brown rice syrup

4–5 sprigs fresh basil, leaves removed, shredded

Preheat oven to 375 degrees.

Place squash and onion in a mixing bowl. Whisk together oil, soy
sauce, orange zest and rice syrup in a small bowl until smooth. Toss with
vegetables to coat. Arrange vegetables in a shallow baking dish, avoiding
overlap. Cover tightly and bake for 45 minutes. Remove cover and return
vegetables to the oven and bake for about 15 minutes, until lightly browned
on the edges. Remove from oven and toss shredded basil gently into the
vegetables, taking care not to break them too much. Transfer to a serving
bowl and serve hot.

PER SERVING: Calories 67; Protein 1.3g; Total Fat 2g; Saturated Fat .24g; Cholesterol 0mg; Carbohydrate 12.5g; Dietary Fiber 3.6g; Sodium 126mg

Roasted Eggplant and Olive Spread

MAKES ABOUT 2 CUPS SPREAD; 8 (¼-CUP) SERVINGS

3 (1-pound) eggplants

2 teaspoons extra-virgin olive oil

4 cloves fresh garlic, crushed

½ teaspoon sea salt

2 teaspoons ground cumin

2 teaspoons white balsamic vinegar

¼ cup finely minced pitted, oil-cured black olives

Preheat oven to 425 degrees.

Pierce eggplants in several places with a fork and lay them on a baking sheet. Bake for about 1 hour, until quite soft. Remove from oven and cool them just enough to handle. Halve the eggplants lengthwise and scoop flesh into a strainer. Allow flesh to drain over the sink for 15 minutes.

Transfer eggplant to a food processor with oil, garlic, salt, cumin, vinegar and olives and puree until smooth. Adjust seasonings to your taste, pulse and transfer to a small serving bowl.

PER SERVING: Calories 74; Protein 2g; Total Fat 2.8g; Saturated Fat .37g; Cholesterol 0mg; Carbohydrate 11.7g; Dietary Fiber 4.5g; Sodium 228mg

Baked Onions with Thyme
MAKES 6 SERVINGS

3 red onions, halved, halves cut into 4 equal pieces
2 yellow onions, halved lengthwise, halves cut into 4 equal pieces
6 cloves fresh garlic, peeled, halved
2 teaspoons extra-virgin olive oil
1 teaspoon sea salt
5–6 sprigs fresh thyme
Zest of 1 lemon, grated
1 tablespoon fresh lemon juice
2 tablespoons fresh thyme leaves

Preheat oven to 375 degrees.

Arrange onions and garlic in a mixing bowl. Toss with oil and salt to coat. Arrange thyme sprigs on the bottom of a shallow baking dish. Arrange onions on top, avoiding overlap. Sprinkle with lemon zest. Cover tightly and bake for 45 minutes. Remove cover and return to oven and bake for about 15 minutes to lightly brown the onions. Remove from oven and toss onions gently with lemon juice. Discard thyme sprigs. Serve hot, garnished with fresh thyme leaves.

PER SERVING: Calories 56; Protein 1.3g; Total Fat 1.7g; Saturated Fat .24g; Cholesterol 0mg; Carbohydrate 9.6g; Dietary Fiber 1.9g; Sodium 387mg

Braised Endive and Pear Slices with Lemon

MAKES 4 SERVINGS

2 teaspoons extra-virgin olive oil

2 teaspoons balsamic vinegar

1 teaspoon sea salt

4 Belgian endive, bottom trimmed, halved

2 ripe, but firm pears (Bosc or red are best)

2 teaspoons fresh lemon juice

Heat oil, vinegar and salt in a flat-bottomed skillet over medium heat. Lay endive, cut sides down, in the pan. Cover; reduce heat to medium-low and cook until the endive wilts and the cut sides brown, about 20 minutes. When the endive is about 80% cooked, halve pears and cut each half lengthwise into thin slices. Lay pears on top of endive, cover and cook for 5 minutes more. Remove from heat, arrange endive halves, cut sides up, with pears laced through the dish. Drizzle with lemon juice. Serve hot.

PER SERVING: Calories 72; Protein .79g; Total Fat 2.6g; Saturated Fat .34g; Cholesterol 0mg; Carbohydrate 12.6g; Dietary Fiber 2.8g; Sodium 586mg

Grilled Fennel and Leeks with Ginger-Miso Sauce

MAKES 4 TO 5 SERVINGS

2 small leeks, split lengthwise, rinsed free of dirt, halved crosswise

1 medium fennel bulb, trimmed, 2 tablespoons coarsely chopped fronds
    reserved, bulb cut into 8 wedges

2 teaspoons avocado oil

¼ teaspoon sea salt

3 cloves fresh garlic, crushed

¼ cup mirin or white wine

¼ cup spring or filtered water

¼ cup sweet white miso

2 tablespoons fresh lemon juice

Place a lightly oiled grill pan over medium heat.

While the grill heats, toss leeks and fennel with oil and ¼ teaspoon salt to coat. Arrange vegetables on grill pan and cook, turning frequently, until just tender, about 12 to 15 minutes.

While the vegetables grill, whisk together garlic, mirin and water in a saucepan and place over medium heat. Simmer for 5 minutes. Remove a small amount of hot liquid and stir in miso until dissolved. Stir miso mixture back into sauce and cook, stirring, for 3 minutes. Do not boil. Remove from heat and whisk in lemon juice.

To serve, arrange grilled veggies on a platter and spoon sauce over top. Garnish with fennel fronds.

PER SERVING: Calories 138; Protein 3g; Total Fat 3g; Saturated Fat .29g; Cholesterol 0mg; Carbohydrate 22.5g; Dietary Fiber 2.8g; Sodium 654mg

Artichoke, Carrot and Zucchini Salad with Lime Vinaigrette

MAKES 5 TO 6 SERVINGS

Lime Vinaigrette
1 jalapeño chile, roasted over an open flame, peeled, seeded and finely
    minced (see Variation, page 217)
5–6 tablespoons fresh lime juice
5–6 sprigs flat-leaf parsley, finely minced
Generous pinch sweet paprika
Generous pinch cracked black pepper
½ cup vegan mayonnaise
1 tablespoon Dijon mustard
¼ teaspoon sea salt

1 cup finely shredded green cabbage
2 cups baby arugula, rinsed well
2–3 sprigs basil, leaves removed, left whole
1 medium carrot, cut into long ribbons with a peeler
1 medium zucchini, cut into long ribbons with a peeler

8 canned artichoke hearts (in water, not oil), halved

10–12 cherry or grape tomatoes, halved

Prepare the dressing: Whisk all ingredients together, adjusting salt to your taste. Cover and refrigerate for 30 minutes before using. Whisk again before mixing with the salad.

Combine all vegetables in a mixing bowl. Just before serving, toss with dressing to coat. Serve immediately.

Variation: You can eliminate the chile from this recipe for a sweeter, less spicy version of the dressing.

PER SERVING: Calories 152; Protein 2.3g; Total Fat 11.3g; Saturated Fat 1.7g; Cholesterol 0mg; Carbohydrate 12.8g; Dietary Fiber 2.6g; Sodium 420mg

Cucumber-Radish Slaw
with Mint Vinaigrette
MAKES 5 TO 6 SERVINGS

2 large cucumbers (English are best here), halved lengthwise, very thinly sliced on the diagonal

8–10 red radishes, halved, very thinly sliced (should be close to 1 cup when sliced)

½ red onion, halved lengthwise, cut into very thin half-moon slices

1 cup very fine julienne or matchsticks fresh daikon

½ teaspoon sea salt

Mint Vinaigrette

3 tablespoons red wine vinegar

2 tablespoons grated orange zest

2 tablespoons finely chopped fresh mint leaves

1 tablespoon fresh lemon juice

2–3 scallions, finely minced

¼ cup extra-virgin olive oil

½ teaspoon sea salt

Generous pinch cracked black pepper

Combine vegetables in a medium bowl. Toss with salt, rubbing the salt into the vegetables with your fingers as you mix. Lay a plate on top of the vegetables, with a light weight on top of the plate (like a large can of tomatoes or a quart of fruit juice). Press vegetables for 15 to 20 minutes. Gently squeeze vegetables between your fingers to expel any remaining fluids and transfer to another bowl. Discard any liquid that accumulated in the bowl while pressing. Lightly rinse the salad if it tastes salty.

While the vegetables press, prepare the vinaigrette: Whisk all ingredients together in a small bowl until emulsified.

To serve, toss vegetables with dressing and serve immediately.

PER SERVING: Calories 132; Protein 1.2g; Total Fat 11.5g; Saturated Fat 1.6g; Cholesterol 0mg; Carbohydrate 7g; Dietary Fiber 1.9g; Sodium 471mg

Pan-Braised Tomatoes with Garlic and Parsley

MAKES 4 SERVINGS

2 tablespoons extra-virgin olive oil

Scant pinch chili powder

Scant pinch ground saffron

⅔ teaspoon sea salt

4 ripe, but firm large plum tomatoes, halved, do not peel or seed

8 cloves fresh garlic, peeled, left whole

5–6 sprigs fresh flat-leaf parsley, coarsely chopped

Heat oil, chili powder, saffron and salt in a flat-bottomed skillet over medium heat. Stir to combine ingredients and lay tomatoes, cut sides down, in the oil. Wedge garlic cloves between tomato halves, cover and listen for a strong sizzle. When you hear it, reduce heat to low and cook until the tomato skins are shriveling and the bottoms are beginning to brown at the edges, 12 to 15 minutes. Transfer tomatoes and garlic to a serving platter, with tomatoes cut-sides up. Sprinkle with parsley and serve immediately.

PER SERVING: Calories 85; Protein .94g; Total Fat 7.2g; Saturated Fat 1g; Cholesterol 0mg; Carbohydrate 4.9g; Dietary Fiber .84g; Sodium 387mg

Tomato and Bread Salad with Roasted Red Onion

MAKES 5 TO 6 SERVINGS

1 red onion, halved lengthwise, cut into thin half-moon slices

2 cups green beans, ends trimmed, left whole

1 cup asparagus tips

3 tablespoons extra-virgin olive oil

1 teaspoon sea salt

10–12 cherry tomatoes, halved

1 cup small-dice cucumbers

1 cup cooked or canned cannellini beans (if using canned, rinse well)

3 cups baby arugula

3 cups 1-inch whole grain bread cubes

2 cloves fresh garlic, crushed

1 tablespoon balsamic vinegar

2 teaspoons fresh lemon juice

3–4 sprigs basil, leaves removed, finely shredded

Preheat oven to 425 degrees.

Toss red onion, green beans and asparagus tips with 1 tablespoon of the oil and ½ teaspoon of the salt to coat. Spread vegetables on a shallow baking sheet and bake, stirring often, until tender and lightly browned at the edges, 12 to 15 minutes. Set aside to cool to room temperature.

Combine tomatoes, cucumbers, cannellini beans, arugula and bread cubes in a large bowl. Whisk together remaining 2 tablespoons oil, remaining ½ teaspoon salt, garlic, vinegar, lemon juice and basil until emulsified.

To serve, gently toss roasted vegetables and dressing into tomato mixture and allow to marinate for about 30 minutes before serving, to soften the bread a bit.

PER SERVING: Calories 217; Protein 6g; Total Fat 9.7g; Saturated Fat 1.4g; Cholesterol 0mg; Carbohydrate 27g; Dietary Fiber 5.8g; Sodium 583mg

Prune, Orange, Fennel and Red Onion Salad

MAKES 4 SERVINGS

1 cup dried pitted prunes, coarsely chopped

½ cup fresh orange juice

Sea salt

2 tablespoons extra-virgin olive oil

1 teaspoon balsamic vinegar

Generous pinch cracked black pepper

2 oranges

1 medium fennel bulb, trimmed, 2 teaspoons chopped fronds reserved,
    bulb halved lengthwise, then cut crosswise into very thin slices

1 red onion, halved lengthwise, cut into very thin half-moon slices

1 small cucumber, halved lengthwise, cut into very thin half-moon slices

5 cups baby spinach or other baby greens

Place the prunes, orange juice and a pinch of salt in a saucepan over low heat. Simmer until prunes are soft, 5 to 6 minutes. Drain, reserving juice, and set prunes aside to cool.

Whisk together oil, vinegar, ½ teaspoon sea salt, pepper and reserved cooking juice from prunes until emulsified. Set aside.

Using a sharp knife, cut peel and white pith from oranges. Catching the juice in a bowl, cut between the membranes to release the orange segments. Reserve the juice for another recipe.

Combine orange segments with fennel, red onion, cucumber and spinach. Toss salad with prunes and dressing to coat the leaves. Serve garnished with fennel fronds.

PER SERVING: Calories 255; Protein 4.4g; Total Fat 7.7g; Saturated Fat 1g; Cholesterol 0mg; Carbohydrate 47.6g; Dietary Fiber 8.7g; Sodium 448mg

Chickpea Puree and Fennel Salad

MAKES 5 SERVINGS

Chickpea Puree

2 cups cooked or canned chickpeas (if using canned, rinse well)

¼ cup finely chopped red onion

2 cloves fresh garlic, finely chopped

2 tablespoons extra-virgin olive oil

1 tablespoon fresh lemon juice

½ teaspoon sea salt

½ teaspoon ground saffron

Spring or filtered water

Fennel Salad

1 small fennel bulb, halved lengthwise, very thinly sliced

1 medium carrot, shaved into long thin ribbons with a peeler

2–3 scallions, cut into 1-inch pieces

1 medium cucumber, cut into julienne pieces

4 cups shredded escarole

1 tablespoon extra-virgin olive oil

1 tablespoon pure flax oil

1 tablespoon fresh lemon juice

2 teaspoons brown rice syrup

⅔ teaspoon sea salt

5 tablespoons pine nuts, lightly pan-toasted (optional)

Make Chickpea Puree: Place all ingredients in a food processor and puree until smooth, slowly adding small amounts of water to create a smooth, thick puree. Set aside.

Make Fennel Salad: Combine vegetables in a large bowl. Whisk together oils, lemon juice, syrup and salt in a small bowl until emulsified. Toss salad with dressing to coat.

To serve, arrange equal portions of salad on 5 plates and top with chickpea puree, dividing equally among the salads. Garnish with pine nuts (if using). Serve immediately.

PER SERVING: Calories 237; Protein 7.3g; Total Fat 12.7g; Saturated Fat 1.6g; Cholesterol 0mg; Carbohydrate 24.2g; Dietary Fiber 7.6g; Sodium 574mg

Tomato Salad with Mint

MAKES 4 TO 5 SERVINGS

3 large ripe, but firm, tomatoes, coarsely chopped; do not peel or seed
½ red onion, cut into very thin half-moon slices
1 cup cooked or canned chickpeas (if using canned, rinse well)
½ cup finely chopped fresh mint
3 tablespoons extra-virgin olive oil
1 tablespoon balsamic vinegar
⅔ teaspoon sea salt
Generous pinch cracked black pepper

Combine tomatoes, red onion, chickpeas and mint in a bowl. Whisk together oil, vinegar, salt and pepper. Gently toss salad with dressing to coat and set aside to marinate for 30 minutes before serving, to make tomatoes easier to digest.

PER SERVING: Calories 180; Protein 4.5g; Total Fat 11.6g; Saturated Fat 1.5g; Cholesterol 0mg; Carbohydrate 15g; Dietary Fiber 3.8g; Sodium 388mg

Leaves of Life

Growing toward the sun with delicate leaves waving in the breeze, these veggies create flexible energy in your body. Too esoteric for you? How about the fact that they are rich in chlorophyll, which aids your body in the production of healthy red blood cells? These seemingly delicate leaves provide you with vascular strength; improve circulation, are rich in essential nutrients and make you feel happy and refreshed.

Stir-Fried Bok Choy with Ginger and Garlic

MAKES 5 TO 6 SERVINGS

1 tablespoon avocado oil

4 cloves fresh garlic, crushed

1-inch piece fresh ginger, cut into fine julienne pieces

Scant pinch crushed red pepper flakes

Soy sauce

½ red onion, cut into thin half-moon slices

1 cup fine julienne pieces fresh daikon

5 baby bok choy, quartered lengthwise, rinsed free of dirt

2 teaspoons black sesame seeds, lightly pan-toasted

Heat oil in a wok or large skillet over medium heat. Add garlic, ginger, red pepper flakes and a splash of soy sauce and stir-fry for 1 minute. Stir in red onion and a splash of soy sauce and stir-fry for 2 minutes. Stir in daikon and a splash of soy sauce and stir-fry for 1 minute. Stir in bok choy and 1 teaspoon soy sauce and stir-fry until wilted, but bright green in color, about 3 minutes. (Add a small amount of water if the vegetables start to stick, but if you stir constantly, you should not need this.)

To serve, arrange vegetables on a platter and sprinkle with sesame seeds.

PER SERVING: Calories 109; Protein 8.4g; Total Fat 4.4g; Saturated Fat .54g; Cholesterol 0mg; Carbohydrate 13.9g; Dietary Fiber 5.8g; Sodium 409mg

Garlicky Collard Greens

MAKES 5 TO 6 SERVINGS

2 tablespoons extra-virgin olive oil

6 cloves fresh garlic, crushed

1 medium yellow onion, halved lengthwise, cut into thin half-moon slices

Sea salt

2 red bell peppers, roasted (see Note, page 153), sliced into ribbons

1 medium bunch collard greens, stem tips trimmed, left whole (see Note,
    page 224)

Place oil, garlic and onion in a large skillet over medium heat. When the onion begins to sizzle, add a pinch of salt and sauté until translucent, about 3 minutes. Stir in bell peppers and a pinch of salt and sauté for 1 minute. Just before adding them to the skillet, slice collard greens into bite-size pieces. Stir into skillet, season with 2/3 teaspoon salt and sauté until wilted and a bright green color, 4 to 6 minutes. Transfer to a serving platter and serve immediately.

Note: Cutting greens ahead of time will result in a loss of nutrients. Cutting them just before cooking allows them to hold on to more of their valuable vitamins. When steaming or boiling, cook them whole and then slice into bite-size pieces after cooking.

PER SERVING: Calories 97; Protein 2.6g; Total Fat 6g; Saturated Fat .84g; Cholesterol 0mg; Carbohydrate 10g; Dietary Fiber 3.9g; Sodium 375mg

Bitter Greens Salad
with Flax-Shallot Vinaigrette
MAKES 5 TO 6 SERVINGS

Flax-Shallot Vinaigrette
3 tablespoons extra-virgin olive oil
1 teaspoon pure flax oil
1 teaspoon brown rice syrup
1 shallot, very finely minced
1 clove fresh garlic, very finely minced
1 tablespoon red wine vinegar
⅔ teaspoon sea salt
Generous pinch cracked black pepper

Bitter Greens Salad
2 Belgian endive, halved lengthwise, sliced into long ribbons
2 cups hand-shredded escarole
2 cups baby arugula
1 cup hand-shredded watercress
1 cup finely shredded radicchio

½ cup coarsely chopped walnuts, lightly pan toasted (optional)

Make vinaigrette: Whisk together ingredients in a small bowl until emulsified. Set aside for flavors to develop.

Make salad: Combine all salad ingredients in a large bowl. Toss gently with dressing to coat the leaves.

Serve immediately with walnuts on the side for those who want a bit of crunch with their salad.

PER SERVING without walnuts: Calories 73; Protein 1g; Total Fat 6.7g; Saturated Fat .94g; Cholesterol 0mg; Carbohydrate 2.8g; Dietary Fiber 1.4g; Sodium 319mg

Tangy Pear and Blueberry Salad
MAKES 4 TO 5 SERVINGS

2 tablespoons pure flax oil

1 tablespoon white balsamic vinegar

1 teaspoon Dijon mustard

½ teaspoon brown rice syrup

2 teaspoons fresh lemon juice

½ teaspoon sea salt

Generous pinch cracked black pepper

2 cups hand-shredded butter lettuce

2 cups hand-shredded watercress

2 cups hand-shredded escarole

2 pears, halved lengthwise, cored and thinly sliced

1 cup fresh blueberries, rinsed well

Whisk together oil, vinegar, mustard, syrup, lemon juice, salt and pepper in a small bowl until emulsified. Set aside while preparing salad ingredients so the flavors of the dressing can develop.

Combine salad greens with pear slices and blueberries in a large bowl. Toss gently with dressing to coat the leaves. Serve immediately.

PER SERVING: Calories 139; Protein 1.7g; Total Fat 7.7g; Saturated Fat 1g; Cholesterol 0mg; Carbohydrate 18.3g; Dietary Fiber 3.9g; Sodium 336mg

Mushroom and Endive Salad

MAKES 3 LARGE SALADS OR 6 SMALLER ONES

1 tablespoon avocado oil

2 cups thinly sliced fresh shiitake mushrooms

½ teaspoon soy sauce

½ teaspoon brown rice syrup

3 Belgian endive, halved lengthwise, thinly sliced crosswise

1 red onion, halved lengthwise, cut into very thin half-moon slices

1 tablespoon extra-virgin olive oil

1 tablespoon pure flax oil or chia seed oil

2 teaspoons red wine vinegar

⅔ teaspoon sea salt

Generous pinch cracked black pepper

Scant pinch chili powder

Heat avocado oil in a skillet over medium heat. Add mushrooms and sauté until they begin to wilt, about 2 minutes. Whisk together soy sauce and syrup and stir into mushrooms. Cook, stirring, until mushrooms begin to brown at the edges, 7 to 10 minutes. Set aside to cool.

Combine endive and onion in a large bowl. Whisk together olive oil, flax oil, vinegar, sea salt, black pepper and chili powder in a small bowl until emulsified. Toss gently with salad to coat the leaves. To serve, mound salad on individual plates and spoon mushrooms equally over top.

Note: If you use chia oil in the dressing, sprinkle chia seeds on top of each salad. Both the oil and seeds are excellent sources of omega-3 fatty acids.

PER SERVING: Calories 162; Protein 2.6g; Total Fat 14g; Saturated Fat 1.7g; Cholesterol 0mg; Carbohydrate 7.8g; Dietary Fiber 2.2g; Sodium 572mg

Mâche Salad with Creole Vinaigrette

MAKES 4 TO 5 SERVINGS

Creole Vinaigrette

1 tablespoon Creole mustard or any spicy hot, smooth mustard

2 tablespoons white balsamic vinegar

½ teaspoon hot pepper sauce

½ teaspoon sea salt

Generous pinch cracked black pepper

¼ cup extra-virgin olive oil

Mâche Salad

1 pound (about 8 cups) mâche (lamb's lettuce)

7 to 8 red radishes, halved lengthwise, very thinly sliced

3 to 4 scallions, thinly sliced on the diagonal

Make vinaigrette: Whisk all ingredients together in a small bowl until emulsified.

Make salad: Combine mâche, radishes and scallions in a large bowl. Just before serving, gently toss with dressing to just coat the leaves. Serve immediately.

Note: Mâche is a salad green with velvety leaves and tender shoots. Often found growing wild, mâche is cultivated in the United States, France and Holland and is rich in vitamin C and B vitamins, including folate. One serving is said to provide 95% of the vitamin C we need in a day, giving us lots of energy and reducing stress.

PER SERVING: Calories 170; Protein 3.5g; Total Fat 15.2g; Saturated Fat 2g; Cholesterol 0mg; Carbohydrate 7g; Dietary Fiber 2.4g; Sodium 436mg

Apple, Arugula and Curly Endive Salad with Hazelnuts

MAKES 4 SERVINGS

2 cups baby arugula

2 cups hand-shredded curly endive (also known as frisée)

1 Granny Smith apple, halved lengthwise, cored, thinly sliced; do not peel

3 to 4 scallions, thinly sliced on the diagonal

3 tablespoons pure flax oil

1 tablespoon balsamic vinegar

⅔ teaspoon sea salt

Generous pinch cracked black pepper

Scant pinch ground cinnamon

¼ cup coarsely chopped, toasted hazelnuts

Combine arugula, endive, apple and scallions in a large bowl. Whisk together oil, vinegar, salt, pepper and cinnamon in a small bowl until emulsified. Toss with salad to coat the leaves. Transfer to a serving platter and sprinkle hazelnuts on top. Serve immediately.

PER SERVING: Calories 167; Protein 1.9g; Total Fat 15g; Saturated Fat 1.8g; Cholesterol 0mg; Carbohydrate 7.9g; Dietary Fiber 2.5g; Sodium 391mg

Sauteed Escarole with Fresh Herbs and Pomegranate

MAKES 3 TO 4 SERVINGS

2 tablespoons extra-virgin olive oil

3 cloves fresh garlic, crushed

1 medium red onion, halved lengthwise, cut into very thin half-moon slices

Sea salt

2 stalks celery, thinly sliced on the diagonal

1 medium head escarole, washed very well

Scant pinch ground nutmeg

Seeds from ½ pomegranate (see Note, page 229)

Place oil, garlic and onion in a skillet over medium heat. When the onion begins to sizzle, add a pinch of salt and sauté until translucent, about 3 minutes. Stir in celery and a pinch of salt and sauté for 1 minute. Hand-shred escarole leaves into bite-size pieces and stir into skillet. Season with ⅔ teaspoon salt and nutmeg and sauté until just wilted, 3 to 5 minutes. Remove from heat and stir in pomegranate seeds. Serve immediately.

Note: To remove the seeds (actually seed sacs, called arils) from a pomegranate, cut a cross in the top of the pomegranate with a sharp knife. Pull the pomegranate into quarters. Submerge the pomegranate in a bowl of cold water. This prevents the pomegranate from staining your fingers. Separate the light-colored membranes and the seeds. The membranes will float and the seeds will sink.

PER SERVING: Calories 153; Protein 3.2g; Total Fat 9.9g; Saturated Fat 1.4g; Cholesterol 0mg; Carbohydrate 15.3g; Dietary Fiber 6.6g; Sodium 661mg

Watercress and Avocado Salad with Basil Vinaigrette
MAKES 4 TO 5 SERVINGS

2 bunches fresh watercress, hand-shredded

½ red onion, cut into very thin half-moon slices

⅓ cup fresh or frozen corn kernels, blanched for 30 seconds

1 ripe, but firm avocado, peeled, seeded and sliced

1 tablespoon fresh lemon juice

Basil Vinaigrette

4 tablespoons extra-virgin olive oil

1 teaspoon Dijon mustard

1 tablespoon fresh lemon juice

½ teaspoon brown rice syrup

½ teaspoon sea salt

Generous pinch cracked black pepper

¼ cup finely shredded fresh basil leaves

2 oranges, peeled and segmented

Combine watercress, red onion and corn in a bowl. Lay avocado slices on a plate and drizzle with lemon juice to preserve color.

Make vinaigrette: Whisk together all ingredients in a small bowl until emulsified.

To serve, arrange salad on a platter. Arrange avocado and orange segments on top and spoon vinaigrette over the whole salad. Serve immediately.

PER SERVING: Calories 262; Protein 3g; Total Fat 22g; Saturated Fat 3.2g; Cholesterol 0mg; Carbohydrate 16.7g; Dietary Fiber 5.3g; Sodium 338mg

Frisée, Escarole and Dulse Salad with Ginger-Wasabi Vinaigrette
MAKES 4 TO 5 SERVINGS

Ginger-Wasabi Vinaigrette
1 tablespoon soy sauce
¼ cup fresh lime juice
1 teaspoon brown rice syrup
2 teaspoons wasabi powder, mixed with just enough water to make a thick paste (see Note, page 231)
2 teaspoons fresh ginger juice
1 tablespoon avocado oil
1 teaspoon sesame oil
2 teaspoons pure flax oil
3–4 scallions, finely minced

Frisée, Escarole and Dulse Salad
2 cups hand-shredded frisée (also known as curly endive)
2 cups hand-shredded escarole
1 cup finely shredded radicchio
1 small cucumber, cut into fine julienne pieces
½ cup dulse fronds, sorted and finely shredded

¼ cup coarsely chopped walnuts, pan-toasted

Make vinaigrette: Whisk together ingredients in a small bowl until emulsified. Set aside for flavors to develop while making the salad.

Make salad: Combine all ingredients, except walnuts, in a large bowl. Toss gently with dressing to coat the leaves.

Transfer to a serving platter and sprinkle with walnuts.

Note: To boost the heat in wasabi, mix it with enough water to create a paste. Place it on a glass saucer and turn a glass or china cup over it to cover. Allow to stand under the glass for 10 minutes. The longer it remains under the glass, the more the heat develops.

PER SERVING: Calories 179; Protein 4.3g; Total Fat 12.6g; Saturated Fat 1.7g; Cholesterol 0mg; Carbohydrate 16g; Dietary Fiber 4g; Sodium 477mg

Garlic-Braised Broccoli
MAKES 4 TO 5 SERVINGS

1 tablespoon extra-virgin olive oil
6 cloves fresh garlic, very finely minced
5 cups ½-inch broccoli florets
½ teaspoon sea salt
¼ cup spring or filtered water

Place oil and garlic in a skillet over medium-low heat. Cook, stirring frequently, for 2 minutes, but do not burn the garlic. Stir in broccoli, salt and water. Cover and increase heat to high. When you hear a strong sizzle, reduce heat to low and cook for 2 to 3 minutes, stirring frequently. Serve immediately.

PER SERVING: Calories 63; Protein 2.9g; Total Fat 3.8g; Saturated Fat .54g; Cholesterol 0mg; Carbohydrate 6.1g; Dietary Fiber 2.7g; Sodium 312mg

Colorful Kale and Pepper Saute

MAKES 4 SERVINGS

2 teaspoons extra-virgin olive oil
½ red onion, cut into thin half-moon slices
Sea salt
½ red bell pepper, roasted (see Note, page 153), cut into thin ribbons
½ yellow bell pepper, roasted (see Note, page 153), cut into thin ribbons
1 medium bunch kale, rinsed well, left whole
2 tablespoons slivered almonds, pan-toasted

Place oil and onion in a skillet over medium heat. When the onion begins to sizzle, add a pinch of salt and sauté until translucent, about 3 minutes. Stir in bell peppers and a pinch of salt and sauté for 1 minute. Just before adding to the skillet, slice kale into bite-size pieces. Stir into skillet, season with ⅔ teaspoon salt and sauté until the kale just wilts and is bright green, about 4 minutes.

To serve, arrange kale and bell peppers on a platter and sprinkle with almonds.

PER SERVING: Calories 102; Protein 4.1g; Total Fat 5.1g; Saturated Fat .57g; Cholesterol 0mg; Carbohydrate 12.4g; Dietary Fiber 2.9g; Sodium 487mg

Spiced Broccoli and Cauliflower

MAKES 4 SERVINGS

Spring or filtered water
Sea salt
1 cup small cauliflower florets
1 medium carrot, sliced into thin coins
1 cup small broccoli florets
2 teaspoons avocado oil
1 teaspoon brown rice syrup
¼ teaspoon ground ginger
¼ teaspoon ground cumin

⅛ teaspoon ground nutmeg
¼ teaspoon chili powder
5–6 scallions, cut into 1-inch pieces

Bring ¾ inch of water to a boil in a deep saucepan with a pinch of salt. Add cauliflower and steam until crisp-tender, about 4 minutes. Remove cauliflower with a slotted spoon. Add carrot to the same water and steam until crisp-tender, about 3 minutes. Remove carrot with a slotted spoon. Add broccoli to the same water and steam until bright green and crisp-tender, about 4 minutes. Mix vegetables together and set aside.

Heat oil and rice syrup in a skillet over medium heat. Stir in ¼ teaspoon salt and spices and cook, stirring constantly, for 3 minutes. Stir in scallions and cook just until they wilt, about 1 minute. Finally, stir in steamed vegetables and cook, stirring until warmed through and coated with spices. Serve immediately.

PER SERVING: Calories 46; Protein 1.6g; Total Fat 2.6g; Saturated Fat .3g; Cholesterol 0mg; Carbohydrate 5.1g; Dietary Fiber 2.2g; Sodium 201mg

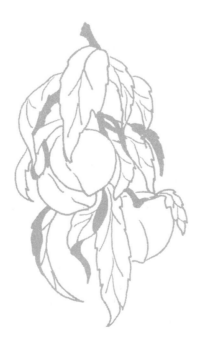

YEAH, DESSERT, BABY!

Change doesn't have to be a drag. Everyone has a sweet tooth and everyone loves a little decadent treat on their tongue. But don't panic; I am not going to tell you to have a bowl of berries, as lovely as they are, when what you want is a bag of cookies.

I think there is a place in a healthy life for dessert, even when you are trying to lose weight. Can you eat huge servings of decadent-tasting sweets every day? Even healthy ones? Nope. Even when a dessert is made from the best-quality ingredients, they are more calorically dense than other foods that you might enjoy in your day, like whole grains and veggies. That said, I know I want to slap those diet gurus who tell me to eat a bowl of steamed kale when I want some dark chocolate. And I love kale! So I can imagine how tough it can be for those of you who are new to kale or may not love it.

Allowing for dessert in your life is just like anything else. At the end of the day, your weight hinges on calories in versus calories out. Period. So how do you have your cake and eat it, too? Well, first you need to grow up and be responsible for what you choose to stuff in your mouth. You have to decide what you really want and then commit to that. And if that commitment includes sweets, then you have to figure out how to handle it so your hips don't expand with each delicious bite. As long as you are committed to regular, vigorous exercise (which burns calories) and as long as you figure the calories of your little dessert (and I mean *little*) into your day, then you will manage your weight without the stress of binge eating.

While you may think of dessert only as an indulgence, the truth is it serves a purpose. Sweet taste is the flavor we crave instinctively. With glucose as the most efficient fuel for your body, is there really any surprise that we gravitate toward anything sweet? So when you attempt to deny your body what it knows it needs, it rebels...in this case, with cravings. It is one of many reasons that diets fail. Such restrictive, boring, not sweet, grim meals will send you right over the edge...fast.

To keep dessert on the menu, there are some basic guidelines that must be put into place for you to succeed. This thinking worked for me and I'm pretty sure it can work for you, too.

Size Matters

Much of the trouble we find ourselves in stems from the fact that we have lost all self-control and with the help of marketing, eat desserts that are sickeningly large in size. After three bites, you really don't taste sweets any-more. Look at European-style desserts. They are generally three to four bite-size tidbits of sweet, just enough to do the trick. You will never see desserts like one restaurant chain's Great Wall of Chocolate Cake, at 2,240 calories a slice. That's your entire day's calories, plus a few hundred extra in just one dessert. Even split four ways, 551 calories are too many for one dessert.

And big-chain restaurants are not the only offenders. You may think you'll just grab one of those giant vegan cookies from your local natural food store. Hang on. These babies can have as much as 350 calories in one giant cookie. Yikes! You have to read the labels and check the ingredients. Sugar is as sugar does. It makes you fat.

Ingredients Are Key

You will find that many (most, actually) vegan desserts that you can purchase are made with sugar (some organic, some not) and unbleached white flour. Your calorie count will be high regardless of the fact that they are vegan. Sure they are made without eggs and milk so you cut some calories and lots of saturated fat, but sugar, sweetened soymilk and vegan margarine replace most of those calories quite nicely, thanks very much.

You want to find desserts with ingredients like organic whole grain flours; unsweetened nut, grain and soy milks; small amounts of good-quality oil for fat and whole, natural sweeteners like brown rice syrup and erythritol (more on that in a bit).

One small caveat here: There's really only one place to find these kind of high-quality desserts: your kitchen, made by your own hand. If you have to make the dessert, you'll enjoy it more, but will be less willy-nilly in your decision to have it because it's on you to create it.

I use organic whole grain flours for my desserts; avocado, olive or Heart Shape flax oil or Earth Balance Spread for my fats; and unsweetened almond milk to replace cow's milk. You can use soy or rice milks as well, but I prefer the results I get with almond milk. Plus, I love the protein, healthy fats and lower calories that are a part of the almond milk package.

Sugar by Any Other Name Is...Sugar

The truth is that simple, refined sugar is completely addictive. It is quickly digested and lands in your bloodstream, altering your blood sugar on impact, so to speak. You get that sensational sugar rush, followed by the inevitable crash. You need more sugar and the cycle of disaster has begun.

Sugar has 194 calories in ¼ cup (that's 4 tablespoons). The average American eats about 133 pounds of sugar each year; that's 500 to 600 calories *each and every day just from sugar.* Not only calorically devastating to any healthy life, sugar also robs the blood of minerals, the bones of calcium and suppresses immune function, making you tired, lethargic and more likely to get and stay sick.

There are other choices to make for sweet living. Brown rice syrup, agave nectar and barley malt top the list, as they are complex carbohydrate sugars, meaning that they digest slowly and don't lead to sugar highs and lows or insulin resistance. Maple syrup and fruit juice are all better for you than sugar (organic or not, raw or not), but they are largely simple sugars, so they also digest quickly and make you crave more.

Of these, brown rice syrup is my personal favorite and the one you will see used most often in my recipes. Its butterscotch flavor is delicate, about half as sweet as sugar, and just great in most of the desserts I make. It has about 170 calories in ¼ cup, so you can see where you can go awry when trying to get control of your caloric intake. Just because it's healthy doesn't mean it has no calories.

However, since starting this book, I have been doing a lot of research. I know that I got myself into trouble with too many desserts even though I was making them from all the "right" ingredients. There had to be alternatives, and of course, there are.

Stevia is an intensely sweet herb whose leaves are ground and powdered for use. Indigenous to South America, stevia is considered by the FDA to be safe for use as a supplement but, oddly, the FDA does not allow it to be marketed as a sweetener. While that thinking is ridiculous, stevia is not my first choice as a low-calorie natural sweetener. Even though it has no calories, 1 teaspoon is equal to 3 cups of sugar in terms of sweetness, which means it is very hard to control the sweetness level. Should you decide that stevia is for you, have at it. You can cook with it, bake with it, stir it into your tea.

Erythritol is my current sweetener of choice. This polyol or sugar alcohol is a natural sweetener made by fermenting naturally occurring plant sugars. While there are several polyol-type sweeteners on the market, this one has stolen my heart and cookie sheets. Unlike some of the other polyols, erythritol is absorbed into the bloodstream in the small intestine, but it is quickly excreted in the urine, so it does not affect blood chemistry at all, nor does it create any stomach distress unless eaten in large amounts.

With about 80% of the sweetness level of sugar, erythritol behaves in cooking and baking much as sugar does, but because it is not absorbed, it has no caloric effect on you. There are some little quirks I have learned in cooking with it to ensure that there is no grainy texture in the final dessert, but that is a small thing compared to how well it does the job of sweetening with no compromise to your health or waistline. In my research I have not found any bad news. And all the experts I have talked to agree. Maybe for once, just once...I hope that I will not eat these words one day. Let's keep everything crossed.

Finally, when you use only the best-quality ingredients like pure extracts, citrus zest and small quantities of nuts and seeds, you ensure that your flavors are interesting as well as sweetly satisfying.

How Many Sweets Can You Enjoy, Really?

I have all sorts of tricks for making desserts now and keeping the portions under control. I collected mini pans for cobblers, cakes and tarts so that I make small desserts and am not tempted by the leftovers. I also freeze pairs of cookies in small snack bags so I enjoy them consciously rather than just sticking my hand into the cookie jar. No doubt you can come up with your own tricks because the real secret is that, when it comes to dessert—any dessert—less is more!

Peanut Butter Cups

MAKES ABOUT 24 PEANUT BUTTER CUPS

2 cups nondairy, grain-sweetened chocolate chips

⅓ cup erythritol

1½ cups creamy, unsweetened peanut butter

1 teaspoon brown rice syrup

½ teaspoon pure vanilla extract

Pinch sea salt

Line the cups of a mini muffin pan with foil candy papers.

Melt the chocolate and erythritol by placing them in a glass bowl over a pan of boiling water and whisk until chocolate and sweetener melt.

Spoon melted chocolate into each cup to fill to one-third. Return remaining melted chocolate mixture to its place over the boiling water, but over low heat, to keep it soft. Place tray in freezer while preparing peanut butter filling.

Combine peanut butter, rice syrup, vanilla and salt in a saucepan and cook over low heat until the mixture is soft and smooth.

Spoon peanut butter on top of each chocolate cup, filling to two-thirds full. Top each cup with remaining melted chocolate, filling the cups full. Place tray in the freezer until set.

PER CUP: Calories 98; Protein 1.3g; Total Fat 6.4g; Saturated Fat 3.2g; Cholesterol 0mg; Carbohydrate 10.6g; Dietary Fiber 1.3g; Sodium 20mg

Apple-Almond Cake

MAKES 10 SERVINGS

2½ cups whole wheat pastry flour

½ cup semolina flour

⅛ teaspoon sea salt

Generous pinch ground cinnamon

Scant pinch ground nutmeg

1 tablespoon baking powder

1 teaspoon baking soda

⅓ cup avocado, olive, or flax-sunflower oil

2 tablespoons brown rice syrup

½ cup erythritol

1 teaspoon pure almond extract

1 cup unsweetened almond milk

1 Granny Smith apple, halved, cored, diced; do not peel

2 tablespoons coarsely chopped almonds

Preheat oven to 350 degrees and lightly oil a standard Bundt pan.

Whisk flours, salt, cinnamon, nutmeg, baking powder and baking soda together. Place oil, syrup and erythritol in a small saucepan and cook over low heat, stirring constantly for 2 minutes. Do not boil. Remove from heat and stir in almond extract. Allow to cool for 2 to 3 minutes before proceeding.

Mix wet ingredients into the dry ingredients. Slowly mix in almond milk until a smooth batter forms. Fold in apple and almonds until well incorporated. Immediately spoon batter into the prepared pan. Bake for 35 minutes, until the top of the cake springs back to the touch.

Variation: Bring 4 tablespoons brown rice syrup to a hard, rolling boil and spoon it over the cooled cake to create a glaze.

PER SERVING: Calories 193; Protein 4.5g; Total Fat 8.7g; Saturated Fat .9g; Cholesterol 0mg; Carbohydrate 25.5; Dietary Fiber 3g; Sodium 271mg

Chocolate-Coconut Macaroons
MAKES ABOUT 3 DOZEN

2 cups erythritol

1 teaspoon brown rice syrup

½ cup unsweetened almond milk

6 tablespoons unsweetened cocoa powder

½ teaspoon pure vanilla extract

½ cup unsweetened shredded coconut

3 cups quick-rolled oats

Line 2 baking sheets with parchment or waxed paper. Combine sweeteners, almond milk and cocoa in a saucepan over medium heat and cook, stirring constantly, until smooth and creamy, about 3 minutes. Remove from heat and stir in vanilla, coconut and oats until combined.

Spoon heaping tablespoons of the mixture onto prepared baking sheets. Allow to cool to room temperature or until they set. If you're in a hurry, place them in the refrigerator and they'll be ready in minutes.

Note: These treats freeze beautifully, so make a big batch and freeze them in small bags for when a chocolate craving hits hard.

PER COOKIE: Calories 31; Protein 1g; Total Fat 1g; Saturated Fat .49g; Cholesterol 0mg; Carbohydrate 5g; Dietary Fiber 1g; Sodium 1mg

Steamed Pear Pudding
MAKES 8 SERVINGS

3 tablespoons unsweetened raspberry preserves
2 cups whole wheat pastry flour
2 teaspoons baking powder
½ teaspoon baking soda
⅛ teaspoon sea salt
Generous pinch ground cinnamon
Scant pinch nutmeg
¼ cup avocado, olive, or flax-sunflower oil
½ cup erythritol
2 tablespoons brown rice syrup
1 teaspoon pure vanilla extract
Unsweetened almond milk
1 ripe pear, halved, cored, diced; do not peel
¼ cup coarsely chopped walnut pieces

Lightly oil a 2-quart pudding basin and lid. Be sure to oil all the little crevices so the pudding doesn't stick. Spoon raspberry preserves evenly into the bottom of the basin.

Whisk together flour, baking powder, baking soda, salt, cinnamon and nutmeg. Combine oil, erythritol and syrup in a small saucepan over low heat, stirring constantly, until the erythritol dissolves, about 2 minutes. Set aside to cool to room temperature. Whisk in vanilla.

Mix together oil mixture and dry ingredients until well combined. Slowly stir in enough almond milk, by ¼ cups, to create a smooth batter. (You should need about ½ cup total.) Fold in pear and walnuts to incorporate. Spoon evenly into prepared pudding basin, filling three-fourths full, and seal the lid.

Place in a pan deep enough to hold the basin. Add enough water to half cover the basin. Cover and bring to a boil. Reduce heat to low and cook for 2 hours, checking the water after 1 hour to see if more is needed. For the pudding to cook, the basin has to remain half-covered by water. After 2 hours, carefully remove the pudding basin and allow to stand, undisturbed, for 5 minutes. Remove the cover and allow to stand for 5 minutes.

Lay a plate on top of the open basin and invert so that the pudding drops gently onto the plate. The raspberry preserves will form a glaze that will run down the sides of the pudding.

Note: Using a pressure cooker for this recipe will cut your cooking time by half.

PER SERVING: Calories 190; Protein 3.7g; Total Fat 9.9g; Saturated Fat 1g; Cholesterol 0mg; Carbohydrate 23.7g; Dietary Fiber 3.1g; Sodium 225mg

Chocolate–Peanut Butter Cookies
MAKES ABOUT 2 DOZEN COOKIES

⅓ cup vegan buttery spread (like Earth Balance)

1 cup erythritol

3 tablespoons brown rice syrup

⅓ cup crunchy, unsweetened peanut butter

1 teaspoon pure vanilla extract

1½ cups whole wheat pastry flour

½ cup quick-rolled oats

Pinch sea salt

Scant pinch ground cinnamon (optional)

Unsweetened almond milk, as needed

1 cup nondairy, grain-sweetened chocolate chips

Preheat oven to 350 degrees. Line 2 baking sheets with unbleached parchment paper or silicone baking sheets.

Combine buttery spread, erythritol, syrup and peanut butter in a small saucepan over low heat. Cook, whisking, until smooth and creamy, about 3 minutes. Remove from heat and whisk in vanilla. Set aside to cool to room temperature.

Mix together flour, oats, salt and cinnamon (if using). Mix wet ingredients into dry ingredients to form a spoonable batter. If too thick or dry, add ¼ cup unsweetened almond milk. Fold in chocolate chips until well incorporated into batter.

With wet hands, roll tablespoons of dough into balls and place onto baking sheets. Press a wet fork into each cookie crosswise, creating a crosshatch pattern in the center. Bake for 12 to 15 minutes. Allow cookies to stand on baking sheets for 2 minutes. Transfer to a cooling rack and cool completely.

PER COOKIE: Calories 98; Protein 1.8g; Total Fat 5.8g; Saturated Fat 2.2g; Cholesterol 0mg; Carbohydrate 11g; Dietary Fiber 1.4g; Sodium 27mg

Almond Cantucci

MAKES ABOUT 2 DOZEN COOKIES

2 cups whole wheat pastry flour
½ cup semolina flour
2 teaspoons baking powder
1 teaspoon baking soda
⅛ teaspoon sea salt
⅓ cup avocado, olive, or flax-sunflower oil
½ cup erythritol
3 tablespoons brown rice syrup
1 teaspoon pure vanilla extract
¼ cup unsweetened almond milk
⅓ cup slivered almonds, lightly pan-toasted

Preheat oven to 350 degrees. Line a baking sheet with unbleached parchment paper or silicone baking sheets.

Whisk together flours, baking powder, baking soda and salt. Combine oil, erythritol and syrup in a small saucepan over low heat and cook, whisking, until the erythritol has dissolved, about 2 minutes. Whisk in vanilla. Set aside to cool to room temperature.

Combine oil mixture and dry ingredients. Mix in almond milk to create a stiff dough. Fold in almonds.

Divide dough in half and form 2 equal logs. Lay them side by side on the lined baking sheet, leaving enough space between them for rising. Bake for 25 to 30 minutes, until firm to the touch. Remove from oven and cool on the baking sheet for 3 minutes. Using a serrated knife, slice each log into ¾-inch wedges. Lay the wedges, cut side up on the baking sheet and return cookies to the oven. Bake for 5 minutes, turn to the other side and bake for 5 minutes more to create a crisp texture.

PER COOKIE: Calories 85; Protein 1.8g; Total Fat 4.2g; Saturated Fat .43g; Cholesterol 0mg; Carbohydrate 11g; Dietary Fiber 1.1g; Sodium 102mg

Pignoli Cookies
MAKES ABOUT 18 COOKIES

1 cup whole wheat pastry flour

1 cup semolina flour

2 teaspoons baking powder

⅛ teaspoon sea salt

¼ cup avocado, olive, or flax-sunflower oil

1 cup almond meal (blanched almonds ground into a fine meal)

½ cup erythritol

2 tablespoons brown rice syrup

1 teaspoon almond extract

¼ cup unsweetened almond milk

1 cup pignoli (pine nuts)

Preheat oven to 350 degrees. Line a baking sheet with unbleached parchment paper or a silicone baking sheet.

Whisk together flours, baking powder and salt. Combine oil, almond meal, erythritol and syrup in a small saucepan over medium heat. Cook, stirring, until well combined and smooth, about 3 minutes. Remove from heat and whisk in almond extract.

Stir almond mixture into dry ingredients and mix well. Add almond milk and mix to create a soft, sticky dough. With wet hands, form dough into 1½-inch balls. Place pignoli in a shallow dish and roll each cookie around, covering with pignoli. Arrange on baking sheet, allowing space for cookies to spread slightly. Bake for 18 minutes. The cookies will still be soft when they come out of the oven. Immediately remove from baking sheet and transfer to a cooling rack.

PER COOKIE: Calories 161; Protein 5g; Total Fat 10.3g; Saturated Fat 1.2g; Cholesterol 0mg; Carbohydrate 13.1g; Dietary Fiber 1.8g; Sodium 66mg

Cinnamon-Braised Apples
MAKES 4 SERVINGS

1 tablespoon vegan buttery spread (like Earth Balance)
1 tablespoon erythritol
2 Granny Smith apples (Gala, Fuji and McIntosh are nice here, too), halved, cored; do not peel
1 cup sparkling apple cider
2 cinnamon sticks
Pinch sea salt
⅛ teaspoon ground nutmeg
½ teaspoon pure vanilla extract
Mint leaves, for garnish

Place buttery spread and erythritol in a flat-bottomed skillet over medium heat. Cook, stirring, for 2 to 3 minutes. Lay apples in skillet, cut sides down, and cook until the apples are beginning to brown at the edges, about 3 minutes. Add apple cider, cinnamon sticks, salt, nutmeg and vanilla. Cover, reduce heat and cook until the apples are tender enough to pierce easily with a fork, about 15 minutes. Do not overcook, as the apples will be mushy. Remove from heat and arrange apples, cut sides up, on a platter. Increase heat under skillet to high and deglaze any remaining liquids to form a thick syrup. Remove cinnamon sticks and spoon whatever liquid remains over the braised apples. Garnish with mint leaves and serve.

Note: If a bit of decadence is on your menu with this dessert, serve the apples hot with a small scoop of vanilla nondairy frozen dessert.

PER SERVING: Calories 83; Protein .21g; Total Fat 2.2g; Saturated Fat .62g; Cholesterol 0mg; Carbohydrate 16g; Dietary Fiber 1.3g; Sodium 66mg

Almond Bar Cookies
MAKES 18 (1½ × 3-INCH) BARS

½ cup almond meal (blanched almonds ground into a fine meal)
¼ teaspoon sea salt
1 cup erythritol
1 tablespoon brown rice syrup
1 cup vegan buttery spread (like Earth Balance)
1 teaspoon almond extract
1¼ cups whole wheat pastry flour
1 teaspoon baking powder
½ cup slivered almonds, lightly pan-toasted

Preheat oven to 350 degrees. Lightly oil a 9-inch-square baking dish.

Combine almond meal, salt, erythritol, syrup and buttery spread in a small saucepan over low heat. Cook, stirring, until erythritol has dissolved and spread has melted, about 3 minutes. Remove from heat and whisk in almond extract. Transfer to a mixing bowl.

Whisk dry ingredients into almond mixture and stir until a spreadable batter forms. Fold in almonds. Spread evenly in prepared pan and bake for 25 to 30 minutes. Remove from oven and cool completely in pan before slicing into bars.

PER BAR: Calories 135; Protein 2.3g; Total Fat 11.6g; Saturated Fat 2.7g; Cholesterol 0mg; Carbohydrate 6.1g; Dietary Fiber 1.3g; Sodium 146mg

Cinnamon-Scented Pear Crisp

MAKES 8 SERVINGS

¾ cup whole wheat pastry flour

1 cup erythritol

½ teaspoon sea salt

1 stick (8 tablespoons) vegan buttery spread (like Earth Balance)

2 tablespoons brown rice syrup

1 cup old-fashioned rolled oats

8 pears (like Bosc or red), halved, cored and cut into ½-inch chunks; do not
    peel

1 tablespoon fresh lemon juice

⅔ teaspoon ground cinnamon

Preheat oven to 350 degrees.

Mix together flour, erythritol and salt. Cut in butter spread and 1 table-spoon rice syrup to create a crumbly texture. Add oats and mix with your hands until moist clusters form. Cover and place in freezer while preparing pears.

Toss pears with lemon juice, remaining 1 tablespoon rice syrup and cinnamon to coat. Spread pears in a shallow 13 × 9-inch pan or 2-quart baking dish. Sprinkle with topping to cover completely. Bake for about 45 minutes, until the topping is golden and the pears are bubbling.

PER SERVING: Calories 149; Protein 3g; Total Fat 1.4g; Saturated Fat .1g; Cholesterol 0mg; Carbohydrate 35g; Dietary Fiber 5g; Sodium 144mg

Rustic Apple Tart

MAKES 4 SERVINGS

Crust

1¼ cups whole wheat pastry flour

Pinch sea salt

2 tablespoons vegan buttery spread (like Earth Balance)

Cold spring or filtered water

Filling
1 teaspoon avocado, olive, or flax-sunflower oil
2 tablespoons erythritol
2 Granny Smith apples, halved, cored, thinly sliced; do not peel
Pinch sea salt
⅓ teaspoon ground cinnamon
1 teaspoon brown rice syrup
Grated zest of ½ lemon

Preheat oven to 350 degrees. Line a baking sheet with unbleached parchment paper or a silicone baking sheet.

Make dough for crust: Place flour and salt in a small mixing bowl and cut in buttery spread to create a texture like wet sand. Slowly add water by tablespoons, and mix just until dough comes together. Knead 3 to 4 times just to pull it together. Do not overknead or overmix or you will create a tough dough. Wrap dough in parchment paper and set aside while preparing apples.

Make filling: Place oil and erythritol in a skillet over low heat and cook, stirring for 2 minutes. Stir in apples and salt and increase heat to medium. Sauté for 2 minutes. Add cinnamon, syrup and lemon zest and sauté until apples are just limp, about 5 minutes. Set aside to cool while rolling out the dough.

Roll out dough into a thin 12-inch-round disk. (Do not worry about it being perfectly round.) Spoon apples evenly onto round, leaving about 1-inch edge. Pull up the side of the dough toward the center but leave the center open, showing filling. Pleat the pulled-over dough decoratively to hold it in place. You will have a round tart, with apple filling showing and a pleated crust. Bake for 25 to 30 minutes, until crust is golden and firm to the touch and apples are bubbling. Remove from heat and serve warm or at room temperature.

PER SERVING: Calories 176; Protein 4g; Total Fat 6.1g; Saturated Fat 1.4g; Cholesterol 0mg; Carbohydrate 29g; Dietary Fiber 4.2g; Sodium 123mg

Coconut Flan with Dark Chocolate Sauce
MAKES 6 SERVINGS

Flan
½ cup silken tofu
1 tablespoon brown rice syrup
½ teaspoon pure vanilla extract
1 teaspoon coconut extract
⅛ teaspoon sea salt
2 tablespoons erythritol
2½ cups unsweetened almond milk
2 tablespoons agar flakes

Dark Chocolate Sauce
1 cup nondairy, grain-sweetened chocolate chips
½ teaspoon pure vanilla extract
Pinch sea salt
Scant pinch ground cinnamon
3 tablespoons erythritol
¼–⅓ cup unsweetened almond milk

Fresh berries and mint leaves when in season, for garnish (optional)

Make flan: Place tofu, syrup and extracts in a blender and puree until smooth.

Combine salt, erythritol, almond milk and agar flakes in a saucepan over medium heat and whisk well. Bring to a boil, stirring constantly. Reduce heat to low and cook, stirring frequently, until agar dissolves, 7 to 10 minutes. Pour hot almond milk mixture into blender with tofu and puree until smooth.

Lightly oil 6 (3-inch) custard ramekins. Pour almond milk mixture from blender evenly into each mold, filling full. Set aside to cool to room temperature. Cover and refrigerate until set, about 30 minutes.

Make chocolate sauce: Place chocolate and vanilla in a heat-resistant bowl and set aside. Combine salt, cinnamon, erythritol and almond milk (using the larger amount for a thinner sauce) in a saucepan and whisk until smooth. Cook over high heat until the mixture comes to a high, rolling boil. Pour over chocolate and whisk until smooth.

Unmold the flans: Dip the bottom of each cup in very hot water; run a sharp knife around the rim and invert onto a dessert plate. Spoon chocolate sauce over top of flans, letting it run down the sides. Garnish with berries and mint (if using).

PER SERVING: Calories 172; Protein 1.7g; Total Fat 9.4g; Saturated Fat 5.7g; Cholesterol 0mg; Carbohydrate 23g; Dietary Fiber 1.9g; Sodium 85mg

Indian Rice Pudding
MAKES 8 SERVINGS

4 cups unsweetened almond milk

4 tablespoons erythritol

1 tablespoon brown rice syrup

1 teaspoon pure vanilla extract

½ teaspoon saffron threads soaked in 2 tablespoons hot water

1 teaspoon ground cardamom

Pinch sea salt

2 cups cooked basmati rice

½ cup golden raisins, plumped in about 1 cup warm water (see Note, page 250), drained and ½ cup soaking water reserved

Garnish

2 teaspoons ground cinnamon

2 teaspoons slivered almonds

2 teaspoons coarsely chopped, shelled, unsalted pistachios

Combine almond milk, erythritol, syrup, vanilla, saffron with soaking water, cardamom and salt in a heavy saucepan over medium heat. Whisking constantly, bring to a boil. Stir in rice, raisins and reserved raisin water, and return to a boil. Reduce heat to very low, cover and cook, stirring frequently, until the pudding is quite creamy and thick, about 35 minutes.

While the pudding cooks, make the garnish: Combine cinnamon, almonds and pistachios in a small skillet over medium heat. Cook, stirring, until the nuts are fragrant, about 4 minutes.

To serve, spoon rice pudding into dessert cups and garnish with toasted nuts.

Note: Plump raisins by soaking them in warm water for about 30 minutes before using. This softens them and draws out some of the excess sugar.

PER SERVING: Calories 150; Protein 2.1g; Total Fat 1.8g; Saturated Fat .3g; Cholesterol 0mg; Carbohydrate 20.4g; Dietary Fiber 1.6g; Sodium 92mg

Mini Pumpkin Cupcakes
with Orange Glaze
MAKES 24 CUPCAKES

2 cups whole wheat pastry flour
½ cup semolina or quinoa flour
2 teaspoons baking powder
1 teaspoon baking soda
⅛ teaspoon sea salt
⅓ teaspoon ground cinnamon
⅛ teaspoon ground nutmeg
¼ cup avocado, olive, or flax-sunflower oil
½ cup erythritol
2 tablespoons brown rice syrup
1 cup canned pumpkin or pureed winter squash
1 teaspoon pure vanilla extract
1 cup unsweetened almond milk
⅓ cup coarsely chopped walnuts

Orange Glaze
½ cup unsweetened orange marmalade
4 tablespoons brown rice syrup

Preheat oven to 350 degrees. Lightly oil a 24-cup mini muffin pan or line with paper liners.

Whisk together flours, baking powder, baking soda, salt and spices. Set aside.

Combine oil, erythritol, syrup, pumpkin and vanilla in a small saucepan. Cook, stirring, until ingredients are smooth and creamy and erythritol is dissolved, about 3 minutes.

Combine the pumpkin mixture with dry ingredients. Slowly stir in almond milk to create a smooth batter. Fold in walnuts. Spoon mixture evenly into muffin cups, filling two-thirds full. Bake until the tops of the muffins spring back to the touch, about 25 minutes. Remove from oven and cool in the baking pan for 7 to 10 minutes. Carefully remove each cupcake and transfer to a wire rack to cool.

Make the glaze while the cupcakes cool: Bring marmalade and syrup to a rolling boil over medium heat. Slip a sheet of parchment paper under the cooling rack and spoon glaze over each cupcake, letting the glaze run down the sides onto the paper. Allow glaze to set for a few minutes before serving.

PER CUPCAKE: Calories 70; Protein 1.9g; Total Fat 1.3g; Saturated Fat .12g; Cholesterol 0mg; Carbohydrate 22g; Dietary Fiber 1.3g; Sodium 127mg

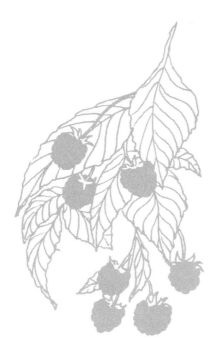

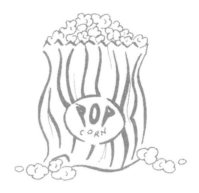

SNACK ATTACK!

The big problem today is that snacks have become feasts, with out-of-control portions, just like all our other food. It's time to get snacks back to sensible little nibbles, not an extension of the meal before. I don't mean with all those silly little packages of artificially flavored, chemical-laced one-hundred-calorie snack bags of sweets. If you're going to take in calories, make them worth it. Know that you are getting a bit of a benefit, as well as satisfaction in the process of snacking.

If you know you are headed to the gym after work, you're going to want a snack that combines protein with some complex carbs so you have energy for your workout. If you have to stay sharp for a meeting, a little healthy fat with veggies will do the trick. If you just want "something," then the world is your oyster.

Most of the snacks in this chapter are savory, but you can also use a bit of one of the desserts in this book to satisfy your mid-afternoon sweet craving.

What I like about these snack options is that they are a lot more satisfying than a few almonds on your way out the door. But make your life easy. Keep a jar of nut butter in your drawer and a bowl of apples on the corner of your desk. When hunger strikes, grab an apple and spread a wee bit of nut butter on some slices for a most satisfying treat. And there's always the option of an ounce of dark chocolate or that handful of nuts to get you through the day. These ideas are for those days when you want and need a little more energy and sustenance.

These snack recipes take a bit of planning and thought, but feeling satisfied all day and not cranky with deprived hunger will be worth it...for you...and everyone around you.

Taco Tarts
MAKES 12 SERVINGS

Cups
24 vegan wonton wrappers
Extra-virgin olive oil

Filling
1 tablespoon extra-virgin olive oil
2 cloves fresh garlic, crushed
¼ red onion, cut into small dice
Sea salt
Generous pinch chili powder
1 stalk celery, cut into small dice
1 cup canned diced tomatoes
1 cup cooked or canned black turtle beans
2–3 scallions, finely diced
1 teaspoon fresh lemon juice

Make cups: Preheat oven to 350 degrees. Lightly oil a 12-cup standard muffin pan. Press one wonton wrapper into each cup, brush lightly with oil and press another on top catty-cornered to the first, forming an 8-pointed cup. Bake for 7 to 10 minutes, until golden brown and crisp. Remove from oven and cool completely before removing from pan.

Make filling: Place oil, garlic and onion in a skillet over medium heat. When the onion begins to sizzle, add a pinch of salt and chili powder and sauté until translucent, about 3 minutes. Stir in celery and a pinch of salt and sauté for 1 minute. Add tomatoes and a pinch of salt and cook for 1 minute. Stir in beans and season with ½ teaspoon salt. Cook, stirring frequently, until the beans are cooked through and mixture has thickened, about 7 minutes. Remove from heat and stir in scallions and lemon juice.

To serve, spoon mixture into the cups. Serve hot or at room temperature.

Note: These freeze beautifully, so make them ahead.

Variation: You can also use prepackaged frozen phyllo cups for this recipe, but the phyllo pastry gets soggy quickly and doesn't hold up as well as the wontons. If using phyllo, serve tarts immediately after filling.

PER SERVING: Calories 76; Protein 2.7g; Total Fat 1.4g; Saturated Fat .21g; Cholesterol 0mg; Carbohydrate 13.8g; Dietary Fiber 1.8g; Sodium 339mg

Hummus and Roasted Pepper Wrap
MAKES 6 SERVINGS (HALF WRAPS)

3 whole grain wraps or soft tortillas
1 (8-ounce) container store-bought hummus
6 leaves romaine lettuce
3 jarred roasted red bell peppers, drained, sliced into thick pieces

Lay wraps on a dry, flat work surface. Spread hummus evenly on each wrap, leaving about ½ inch uncovered around the perimeter. Lay a large lettuce leaf on hummus and top with roasted peppers, dividing evenly. Roll the wraps, jelly-roll style, into tight cylinders. Slice in half and wrap in plastic.

PER SERVING: Calories 137; Protein 5.3g; Total Fat 4.7g; Saturated Fat .63g; Cholesterol 0mg; Carbohydrate 19.5g; Dietary Fiber 3.2g; Sodium 490mg

Avocado and White Bean Dip
MAKES 5 SERVINGS

2 ripe Haas avocados, peeled, coarsely chopped
⅔ cup cooked or canned cannellini beans
⅓ red onion, very finely diced

¼ cup finely chopped fresh basil
2 teaspoons fresh lemon juice
1 teaspoon pure flax oil
⅔ teaspoon sea salt
Generous pinch cracked black pepper

Place avocados in a bowl and mash with a fork until smooth. Fold in beans, onion, basil, lemon juice, oil, salt and pepper, stirring gently until well combined. Serve at room temperature or chilled.

PER SERVING: Calories 168; Protein 3g; Total Fat 13.4g; Saturated Fat 2g; Cholesterol 0mg; Carbohydrate 11.6g; Dietary Fiber 5.5g; Sodium 383mg

Braised Kale Crostini
MAKES 3 SERVINGS

2 teaspoons extra-virgin olive oil
2 cloves garlic, crushed
¼ red onion, cut into thin half-moon pieces
½ teaspoon sea salt
Pinch crushed red pepper flakes
2 cups coarsely chopped kale
3 slices whole grain bread

Place oil, garlic and onion in a skillet over medium heat. When the onion begins to sizzle, add a pinch of the salt and red pepper flakes and sauté until translucent, about 3 minutes. Stir in kale and season with remaining salt. Sauté kale until it wilts and is a deep green, about 3 minutes.

While the kale wilts, toast the bread. Cut toasted slices in half, creating triangles and evenly mound kale mixture on each piece.

PER SERVING: Calories 122; Protein 4.3g; Total Fat 4.4g; Saturated Fat .69g; Cholesterol 0mg; Carbohydrate 18g; Dietary Fiber 2.8g; Sodium 530mg

Guacamole with Roasted Tomatoes and Garlic

MAKES 4 SERVINGS

Roasted Tomatoes
15 cherry tomatoes
7 cloves fresh garlic, peeled, left whole
2 teaspoons extra-virgin olive oil
Pinch sea salt
Pinch cracked black pepper
Pinch dried basil

Guacamole
2 ripe avocados
⅓ cup very finely diced red onion
1 jalapeño chile, very finely diced (do not remove seeds)
3 tablespoons fresh flat-leaf parsley or cilantro
1 tablespoon fresh lemon juice
⅔ teaspoon sea salt
Generous pinch cracked black pepper

Baked chips or veggie sticks, to serve

Preheat oven to 400 degrees.

Make tomatoes: Place tomatoes, garlic, oil, salt, pepper and basil in a plastic bag, seal and toss to coat the tomatoes. Arrange on a baking sheet, avoiding overlap. Bake until the skins begin to pop and wrinkle, about 10 minutes. Remove from oven and cool to room temperature.

Make guacamole: Cut avocados in half, remove seeds and scoop out flesh into a medium bowl. Mash coarsely with a fork. Add remaining ingredients and mix well.

When the tomatoes and garlic are cool enough to handle, chop coarsely and fold into guacamole. Chill for about 1 hour before serving to allow the flavors to develop. Serve with baked chips or veggie sticks.

PER SERVING: Calories 208; Protein 3g; Total Fat 18g; Saturated Fat 2.8g; Cholesterol 0mg; Carbohydrate 13.2g; Dietary Fiber 6g; Sodium 432mg

Maple Popcorn

MAKES 3 TO 5 SERVINGS

⅓ cup brown rice syrup

2 teaspoons maple granules (granulated maple syrup)

2 tablespoons erythritol

1 teaspoon avocado oil

Pinch sea salt

1 teaspoon pure vanilla extract

6 cups air-popped popcorn

3 tablespoons coarsely chopped pecans (optional)

Place syrup, granules, erythritol, oil and salt in a saucepan over medium heat. Whisk briskly and cook until it reaches a rolling boil. Boil for 5 minutes. Whisk in vanilla.

Lightly oil a mixing bowl and place popcorn and pecans (if using) in it. Stir in syrup mixture and toss with an oil-coated spoon (to prevent sticking) until the popcorn is coated. Set aside to cool. When the popcorn is cooled, break off chunks and enjoy.

Variation: Savory Popcorn: Toss the popcorn with 1 tablespoon avocado oil, a pinch of salt and 1 teaspoon chili powder, dried herbs or curry powder.

PER SERVING: Calories 183; Protein 2g; Total Fat 5g; Saturated Fat .5g; Cholesterol 0mg; Carbohydrate 37.9g; Dietary Fiber 2.4g; Sodium 48mg

Power Smoothie

MAKES 2 SMOOTHIES

½ banana

½ cup frozen raspberries

½ cup frozen blueberries

½ teaspoon pure vanilla extract

1 scoop vegan rice protein (see Note, page 258)

1½ cups unsweetened almond milk

Combine all ingredients, except almond milk, in a blender. Blend, slowly adding almond milk to achieve a thick, creamy consistency. Serve chilled.

Note: Vegan rice protein will add some power to this smoothie, but is optional and only needed if you are working out extra hard. Look for one that has few ingredients and no artificial additives. Your best bet is to look for one in a natural food store to get the best quality.

PER SERVING: Calories 129; Protein 7g; Total Fat 3g; Saturated Fat 0g; Cholesterol 0mg; Carbohydrate 20.8g; Dietary Fiber 4.1g; Sodium 6mg

Tomato, Onion and Chile Salsa

MAKES ABOUT 4 CUPS; 12 (⅓-CUP) SERVINGS

4 medium ripe tomatoes, coarsely chopped; do not seed or peel

½ red onion, finely diced

2 serrano chiles, stems, ribs, seeds removed, finely diced (see Note, below)

3 cloves fresh garlic, very finely minced

Juice of 1 lemon

⅔ cup coarsely chopped fresh flat-leaf parsley

⅓ cup coarsely chopped fresh cilantro

⅔ teaspoon sea salt

Generous pinch cracked black pepper

Generous pinch ground cumin

1 teaspoon extra-virgin olive oil

Combine all ingredients in a medium bowl and stir to combine. Cover and set aside for 1 hour before serving to allow flavors to develop, stirring occasionally. Serve with baked chips or as the garnish on tacos, a black bean dish or even on top of a salad.

Note: If you leave the seeds and ribs in the chiles, you may have far more heat than you want.

PER SERVING: Calories 14; Protein .45g; Total Fat .52g; Saturated Fat 0g; Cholesterol 0mg; Carbohydrate 2.3g; Dietary Fiber .54g; Sodium 132mg

Sauteed Mushroom Crostini

MAKES 3 TO 6 SERVINGS

2 teaspoons extra-virgin olive oil

½ yellow onion, cut into small dice

Sea salt

Generous pinch cracked black pepper

½ cup dried maitake mushrooms, soaked until tender, about 5 minutes

3 cups coarsely chopped mixed fresh mushrooms (cremini, button, oyster, morels, portobello)

3 slices whole grain bread

½ cup coarsely chopped fresh flat-leaf parsley

1 teaspoon fresh lemon juice

Place oil and onion in a skillet over medium heat. When the onion begins to sizzle, add a pinch of salt and pepper and sauté until translucent, about 3 minutes. Drain maitake mushrooms, reserving water. Stir all mushrooms into skillet and add a pinch of salt and sauté until mushrooms release their juices and begin to reabsorb them. Season with ½ teaspoon salt and add ⅓ cup of the mushroom soaking water to the skillet (discard the remaining water or use in another recipe). Cover and reduce heat to low. Cook, stirring frequently, until mushrooms are tender and beginning to brown, about 8 minutes.

When the mushrooms are almost ready, toast the bread and cut slices in half, creating triangles. Remove mushrooms from heat and stir in parsley and lemon juice. Spoon evenly onto toast pieces and serve hot.

PER SERVING: Calories 159; Protein 7.6g; Total Fat 4.4g; Saturated Fat .7g; Cholesterol 0mg; Carbohydrate 26.3g; Dietary Fiber 4.1g; Sodium 618mg

NATURAL HOME REMEDIES

Sometimes we need a quick fix for an acute symptom, a jump start to get energy moving or a little concentrated help for a chronic condition. There are lots of over-the-counter products that we're more than willing to spend billions of dollars on to prevent indigestion, get rid of a headache, unstuff a stuffy nose, break up chest congestion, mask our aches and pains, kick-start weight loss, burn fat, get rid of spots and pimples, and diminish wrinkles.

But what if I told you that right in your kitchen you have the ingredients to create gentle remedies to handle many of these same conditions? You won't just mask symptoms and cover flaws; these simple recipes relieve the symptom and help get to the root of the problem, so the symptoms can actually go away. How cool is that?

These few natural remedies are a part of your eating plan to aid you in the process of achieving your ideal weight and creating strong, vital health.

Carrot Daikon Drink

MAKES 1 SERVING

This spicy, pungent tea is designed to help dissolve hardened fat deposits that have accumulated deep within various organs, inhibiting their function. Working deep in the body to restore balance, this drink works to dissolve the fat, while adding minerals to create strong blood quality. This is the remedy to begin your weight-loss process.

Some of the ingredients are a bit exotic, but can be found in most natural food stores. The results are worth the effort of finding the right foods to use in this tea.

½ cup finely grated carrot
½ cup finely grated daikon
1 cup spring or filtered water
Splash soy sauce
⅓ sheet toasted sushi nori, shredded
⅓ umeboshi plum*

Combine grated vegetables with water in a saucepan over medium heat. Bring to a gentle boil, uncovered. Reduce heat to low and simmer, uncovered, 3 to 4 minutes. Add soy sauce and simmer for 2 to 3 minutes more. Stir in shredded nori and umeboshi plum and simmer for 1 minute more. Drink the tea and eat the vegetables, while the tea is quite hot.

Note: You will begin to sweat as you eat the vegetables and drink this tea. It's powerful!

Shiitake Tea
MAKES 1 SERVING

This simple tea is designed to regulate kidney function, softening them so they can do their job efficiently … to detox and aid in weight loss.

1 dried shiitake mushroom
1 cup spring or filtered water
Splash soy sauce

Soak shiitake mushroom in water until tender, about 20 minutes. Finely mince and place with the soaking water in a saucepan over medium heat. Bring to a boil, uncovered. Reduce heat to low and simmer for 10 to 15

---

* Umeboshi plums are pickled, unripened plums sold in natural food stores.

minutes. Add soy sauce and simmer for 2 to 3 minutes more. Drink liquid and eat mushroom, while hot.

Note: This tea can also be quite effective in relaxing overall tension or tightness in the body.

Kombu Tea

MAKES 2 SERVINGS

Kombu tea is an amazing restorative. Kombu has so many benefits in the body: strengthening blood quality; dissolving animal fats, which helps to stimulate the loss of hard fat on our bodies; and balancing nervous system function. That's a lot of power for a simple sea plant.

3-inch piece kombu
4 cups spring or filtered water

Place kombu and water in a saucepan over medium heat. Bring to a boil, covered. Reduce heat to low and simmer until the liquid reduces by half, 10 to 15 minutes. Drink 1 cup while hot. You may reheat remaining tea for another serving.

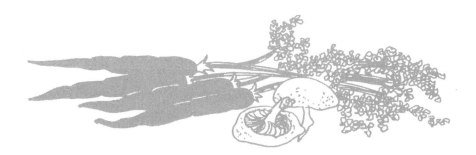

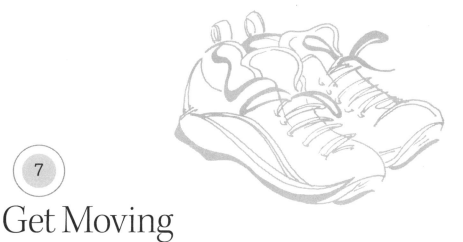

7

Get Moving

The only way to get that fat off is to eat less and exercise
more.   — JACK LALANNE

Exercise is not only about getting thinner. Consider the 2006 study
published in the *Journal of Aging and Health* in which sixty-four people, aged sixty-six to ninety-six were divided into three groups. One
group worked out with resistance training, the second group exercised by
walking and the third group did nothing at all. After exercising only twice
a week for sixteen weeks, both groups who worked out showed lower sys-
tolic blood pressure, improved body strength and flexibility, improvement
in balance and coordination and weight loss.

We all know the benefits of exercise. We read about them ad nauseum.
We see news reports and magazine articles telling us these indisputable
truths. And they are all true. But the biggest truisms are these: It's never
too late to begin and you are never so out of shape that you can't get some
semblance of fitness back. It's time to stop making excuses and get off the
couch.

In chapter 3, "The Path to Rethinking Your Life," I introduced the five
key principles to your total life makeover. In this chapter, I'd like to revisit
the first two principles, Prepare and Make Choices, but with specific ref-
erence to exercise. Without making a conscious effort to prepare and to

make the right choices for you when it comes to exercise, any course you take is unlikely to give the results you'd like to see.

PREPARE

It all starts here. To get and stay motivated, rather than focusing on why you can't, haven't or won't exercise, ask yourself why you want to exercise—not why you *should*, but why you *want* to. Do you want to lose weight? Do you want to be stronger? Do you want to avoid disease? Whether it's one or all of these issues, answering these questions and keeping them uppermost in your thoughts (that's the rethinking part), puts you at your starting point and, as you progress, you'll find that your motivation to achieve the results you want increases, rather than wanes. When your intention is set by determining the reasons you set out on this path, everything will flow from there—with a little help from me and the advice in this book.

Eye on the Prize

A key part of preparation is setting goals for yourself. A lot of experts say that you should set small goals so that you don't set yourself up for failure. They say that you should set short-term goals like walking for twenty minutes on Monday, Wednesday and Friday. They say that this will keep you inspired. I say that we are way past all of that, because it hasn't worked for most of us in the past. We need to get our butts moving and we need to sweat. So set a goal that you may never achieve. If you are walking around the block today, set the goal of a marathon. If you are faithfully performing the exercises in this book, set the goal of attending and finishing a boot camp–style class. Reach for the stars. You may just surprise yourself.

Make Fitness a Habit

Your fitness has to become second nature to you, like washing your face in the morning, like brushing your teeth, like breathing. It has to become a part of your everyday life in order for you to achieve any level of physical strength and endurance. A lot of people struggle with this. They begin their routine with all good intentions (like the ones that pave the road to hell), but get derailed the second something comes up that interferes with their carefully scheduled day. I know that with the busy life I lead, I have to schedule exercise just like I schedule the rest of my day's obligations. When you make an appointment with yourself and write it in your calendar, you are more likely to stick with it. Writing that appointment down makes it real—and as important as anything else in your day. I have made a pact with myself that if it's in the calendar, I drop what I am doing when it's time to exercise.

Yes, there will be days when you are tired, stressed, overworked and you just want to go home, kick off your shoes and drop onto the couch and chill. Instead, lace up your shoes and go for a walk or begin your workout routine, even if you are fighting with yourself to do it. There are days when I drag myself to the gym, thinking that exercising is crazy. What I need is rest, not more work. But I go and within ten minutes of getting on that spin bike; within ten minutes of a run; within ten minutes of working with my trainer, Anthony, I realize that what I needed was exercise. I needed to move my tired body, feel the circulation increase with the stress of the workout. What I needed was the feeling of strength in my muscles as I work, the endorphin rush that allows me to let go of the day and focus on my fitness. I go home spent from the workout, but glowing with the resulting energy. I am literally healed from my busy day at the gym. Of course, you need rest, too, so be sure and plan in one day a week with no working out, just rest.

Making Choices

When I came to the realization that I had to get serious about exercise, I was forty-seven years old and thirty-five pounds heavier than I wanted to be. That may not sound like a lot, but trust me it is just as hard to lose 35 pounds as it is to lose 135. It may take more time to lose more weight, but the choices that I had to make were just the same: what goals should I set for myself? where and how to start? what's the right path for me? But first, I had to rethink exercise and reeducate myself about what's really important.

The Great Triumvirate

Nope, this isn't going to a crash course in the politics of ancient Rome but a simple lesson in the three things that we have to consider as part of a well-balanced exercise program: cardiovascular health, muscular strength and flexibility. Once you understand how important each of these components is to your health and fitness you'll find a renewed motivation to stick with the program.

NO MORE HEART ACHES

Cardiovascular exercise may not save your love life but it is crucial to weight loss and heart health (get it? cardiovascular exercise?). I found that out the hard way…by not doing it and just lifting weights. Instead of lean and fit, I was bulky and fit. Fit and big was not the result I was going for.

You must get your heart rate up to see results. And you don't need a gym to do it. Walking, jogging, speed walking or biking are all easy, portable and can be done anywhere, at any time. All you need is a good pair of shoes (or a bike) and motivation. You can walk in the park, in your neighborhood or walk to complete your errands for the day. Rather than sit at your desk, hunched over a microwaved bowl of junk food, take a twenty-minute walk, three days a week, working out on the alternate days. Eat something fresh and energizing when you get back to the office. You will feel refreshed, relaxed, awake and happy.

But remember, the goal is to raise your heart rate, which means a *brisk* walk, not a meandering stroll. If you want to walk with a friend for inspiration, cool by me. Just make sure that your chatty conversation comes with the effort of breathing hard. Better yet, talk when you get back to the office or home. Walk with a purpose. Make it a workout, not a social visit.

If using machines at a gym make it easier for you to pull this off, then by all means, hit the gym. Personally, the thought of thirty to forty-five minutes on a treadmill or stair machine can make me crazy. I need to get somewhere, do something or I will grow bored and stop. But, hey, if the treadmill does it for you, hit it. But hit it hard. You must change your routine to change your body. And cardio…sweaty, hard, oh-God-it's-hard-to-breathe cardio is the best and most effective way. After a week or two, you will change. The dread that you may now feel about starting an exercise program will soon be replaced with crankiness when you *can't* get it. (This is the only time I'll let you be a junkie…)

STRENGTH TRAINING

The second part of the exercise equation is strength training. (Ah, visions of Arnold S. are dancing in your head…) I know, I know; you don't like this either. Are you seriously worried about bulking up like the Hulk? Have you any idea what it takes to get those bulging, vein-popping muscles? Forget it. It won't happen. Are you are worried about being the weakling at the gym, lifting your five-pound dumbbells next to the muscular dude who could bench-press you? Do you hate the idea of being the unfit slug in a sea of fit, perfect bodies? Forget all that! If you walk your sorry butt into a gym, you will see people just like you who are just getting started and feeling (and looking) just as awkward. And right next to them is the fit and trim specimen of a person who's likely helping and guiding them along, making them feel comfortable in this new situation and not in the least, inspiring them.

But I do understand those feelings. I was there. That's why I designed (with the help of my wonderful trainer, Anthony Molino) an at-home, get-in-shape-now routine that will raise your confidence as well as your fitness, so you can walk into the gym—or anywhere—feeling fitter and stronger. Bring it on, Ah-nold!

But you can fit fitness in anywhere: Stirring a pot of soup on the stove? Do two sets of twelve pliés while you stir and you have just worked out your butt and the backs of your thighs and abs! Yard work—heavy gardening, hauling mulch bags around, mowing the lawn with a push mower, raking leaves vigorously, sweeping the street with energy. All of these simple daily activities work your muscles, making you stronger. (Just don't be a moron and overdo it the first day out…but more about that later.) And as you get stronger, working out will not seem so awful or foreign…and all you are doing is maintaining your everyday life.

Training your muscles does more than prevent your butt from looking like a gang of kids fighting under a blanket as you walk. Strong muscles are essential to strong bones. When you work out with resistance, bone growth is stimulated; muscle cushions and protects your bones. Your skeleton stays strong. No wussy, hunched-over, slumped spine for you!

FLEXIBILITY

Flexibility doesn't mean you have to look like a contortionist with your legs wrapped about your head while you do a handstand. It's one thing to be toned and strong and quite another to have your muscles get so tight that you can't scratch your own head. Gentle stretching helps your muscles to grow lean and long, not bulky and cumbersome. Stretching is also relaxing, and stress reduction is one of the keys to weight loss. From stretching on the floor as you watch television, to yoga and Pilates classes, creating a flexible body is as important as creating a strong one. Stretching eases your mind, opens your body and relaxes your muscles. Stretch for about five minutes every day and you will be hooked...

WHAT'S RIGHT—AND WHAT'S RIGHT FOR YOU

Exercise is hard work, but it should be fun for you, too. And I know you have heard this a million times and then some, but finding an activity you like will make exercise more natural for you and ensure that you stick with it. For many people, there is more than one thing that floats their boat, so they try all sorts of things and settle into a routine. For me, I need the stimulation of variety, so I spin on Monday and Thursday, take a boot camp class on Tuesday, train with Anthony on Wednesday and Friday, and run on Thursday (a split workout day) and Sunday. I take Saturday off from all things fitness, so that my body can recover. Some weeks require that I only work out five days a week, but I love the weeks when I can get in six days of a good sweat.

Many people feel more inspired and motivated in a group setting so don't discount the idea of going to a class a few times a week. I love the camaraderie that comes with group training. When we are all straining on spin bikes, clapping and cheering each other on, that makes it fun and more exciting. I am not so sure that I would work as hard if I were on that spin bike in a room all by myself. On the other hand, I love the solitude that comes with biking on trails here in Philadelphia or running along city streets, challenging and pushing myself to work harder.

If a group is what you need, find a class. If you need inspiration and support, enlist a friend to work out with you. You can alternate and meet at each other's homes, working out and socializing at the same time. Just be sure and work out; don't let your time for fitness turn into a gab fest. Work! This is your fitness time...make other arrangements for coffee and gossip.

Take It Personally

While I am an advocate of using personal trainers I know that it's not an option for everyone. So I am asking that you let this book and me serve as your personal trainer. And I'm asking you to make the same kind of commitment that often comes when you sign up to work with a trainer and pay in advance for a series of sessions. You're motivated by your financial investment and by the trainer, who will keep you inspired. (A good trainer will certainly teach you the proper form and how to adapt a workout to your own needs.) But the best motivation will come from you and your desire to get fit and healthy. After all, it's not the trainer that gets the results—it's your own hard work.

GETTING STARTED

Now's the fun part—getting started. And it's a lot easier than you think. You don't have go out and buy lots of fancy equipment (although a good pair of exercise shoes is vital) so you can't use having to shop as an excuse. "I haven't a thing to wear!" doesn't cut it with me. Everyone's got a pair of shorts and a T-shirt!

Ladies and Gentlemen, Start Your Engines!

Cardiovascular exercise is essential to weight loss and maintenance, so let's get that bit in play immediately. You don't need anything special for cardio; no equipment, no tools. Just a good pair of walking shoes and you can get started. Depending on your current condition, walk around the block. The next day, walk two…and then four and then eight. Build up to walking a mile each day within two weeks, gradually increasing your pace with your distance. When you reach one mile, you should be breathing hard, making conversation difficult. Once you have mastered briskly walking a mile, you can move onto other, more intense cardio workouts. But be realistic. If you haven't exercised in years, it will be difficult at the start to go from zero to working out six days a week. Shoot for three days a week for the first week, with time to recover; then five days a week and then six days a week when you are feeling stronger.

Keep in mind that Rome wasn't built in a day and your return to fitness, while it won't take decades to rebuild, will be a gradual process. You won't progress from walking a few blocks at a brisk pace to a marathon in two weeks. You can certainly build up to that, but it will take time. And in that time, you must stay committed and stay inspired, which will be easy as you begin to notice the changes in your body, strength and endurance.

Strength Training to Beat the Band!

When I began to train with Anthony Molino, we did a lot of exercise using a *resistance band*—you know, those long, brightly colored things that look like somebody took the elastic out of the waistband of your stretchy pants—in place of free weights. Even now, I still use the band on occasion in my training and especially when I travel and there's no gym close by. With the workout we devised below, plus thirty minutes walking and jogging daily, I lost ten pounds and a dress size in three weeks. Three weeks!

Resistance bands are great for improving coordination as well as strength. Since there is tension in all parts of the movement, you need to stabilize your body to do the moves, which improves balance and helps you involve more muscle groups for a more complete workout. I love that anybody can use these bands, from beginners to the seriously fit. They are *real* equipment—and a lot less cumbersome than exercise machines that are of doubtful value. *Prevention* magazine tested a group of otherwise sedentary women using weight training, yoga, Pilates, resistance bands and body-weight exercise, like push-ups. The group using the bands lost 30% more inches off their tummies, hips, arms and thighs, averaging a total loss of fifteen inches over a twelve-week period. They also dropped 18% more weight. They also worked out more because the bands were accessible and easy to use. Cool, huh?

I like to do this workout to upbeat dance music ("The Final Chapter" is my favorite) and keep my reps to the beat. It makes it more of an interval-style workout, keeping my heart rate up, so my cardio extends way past my morning jog. But it's your call. Pop on your iPod; do it while watching Oprah or the news on CNN; do it on the deck or patio to be in the fresh air or do it peacefully, in the quiet, for a zen workout. Just do it.

Oh, and did I mention that this can be a really fun workout to get the kids into? Teach them the routine and let them do it on their own, at their own pace. Or work out together. Instilling a love of fitness in them early in life ensures that they will not become statistics, but will live lives of fitness and health.

Do this full-body workout every other day, for a total of three days a week. It takes about thirty-five minutes to complete two sets of fifteen reps of each of the ten moves. In the beginning, rest for about one minute between sets to let your self recover a bit. But as you grow stronger, try to move smoothly from move to move with minimal rest. This will keep your heart rate revved and you'll burn more fat. (You'll also need to include three to five thirty- to sixty-minute cardio sessions each week for total success. Your brisk walk will work just fine...but remember it has to be brisk (meaning difficult to talk) but not impossible to breathe. (See "Ladies and Gentlemen, Start Your Engines" above.)

I truly think that you will love this workout and it will inspire you to do more...and more...and more.

What You'll Need

Okay, here's your excuse to do a little shopping...You will need a resistance band with handles. You can buy a version without handles, but the ones with the handles are a lot easier to grip and maneuver. They cost about $10 each, so your investment in your fitness is next to nothing. They come in various resistances, from light to heavy, so you'll need to decide how hard you want to work. I personally love the SPRI Xertube (you can find them at any sporting goods store or at www.spriproducts .com). I recommend that you get a light, medium and a heavy band (okay, so it's a $30 investment). I like having a variety of resistances around so that I can use the lighter band for smaller muscle groups and the heavy band for the bigger muscles. Plus the variety of bands allows you to intensify your workout as you see progress. But you know what? You can just buy one to get started.

Read the instructions through before performing each move. Be sure to refer to the "Form" comments on each move to ensure that you get the maximum benefit and avoid injury. Enjoy!

Reverse Lunge

This exercise tones your butt and legs. You will look great from behind in your jeans.

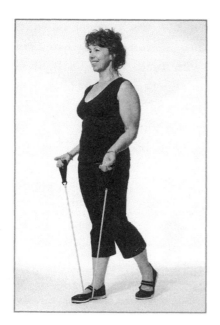
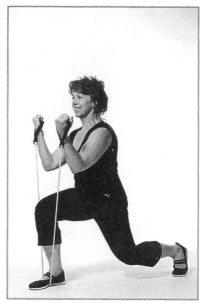

Start: Stand with your left foot 2 to 3 feet in front of your right, with your back heel off the floor. Place your band under your left foot, holding a handle in each hand at shoulder height, palms facing forward. Bend both knees, lowering your hips, keeping your back straight, until your left thigh is parallel with the floor. Hold for 1 count; straighten up, keeping your body straight. Do 1 full set of 15 reps and then repeat on the other leg.

Form: Keep your tummy sucked tightly in, as though trying to get your belly button to touch your spine. When you bend your knees, count 3 seconds as you lower; hold for 1 count and then count 3 seconds as you straighten up. This keeps your form controlled and poised. Breathe out as you lower into the lunge and inhale as you straighten up.

As you get stronger and want to see that excellent definition in your thighs, try this added move. Before each rep, perform 8 mini-pulses, meaning from the start position, you raise up only 2 to 3 inches and lower back to the start. Move at double-time speed.

Side Ab Bend

This works your abdominals and your obliques (side abs, you know, your love handles or muffin-top spot).

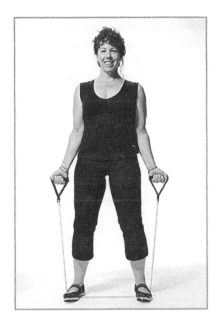 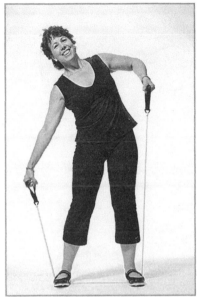

Start: Stand with both feet just slightly wider than hip-width apart. Place the band under both feet, stretched taut equally, handles in each hand. Bend knees slightly. Keeping your chest high, reach your left hand down to your left foot, while bending to the left side. At the same time, lift your right elbow toward your right shoulder. Switch position of arms as you bend to the other side to complete 1 rep. Complete 15 full reps (side bends to right and left sides).

Form: Keep your tummy pulled tightly in and your chest held high. Bend from the side; don't turn as you bend. The motion is like you were sliding your hand down the side of your leg, while facing forward. Do not twist as you bend. Count 3 seconds to the bottom; hold for 1 count and then count 3 seconds to straighten up.

As you get stronger, hold a 3- to 5-pound dumbbell in each hand and add a bit of extra resistance as you bend to the side to really tighten up those side abs.

Shoulder Pull-Down

This exercise works your shoulders, abs, butt and legs, so you look sexy in any-thing…and have the strength to power through your day

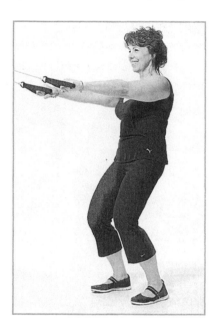
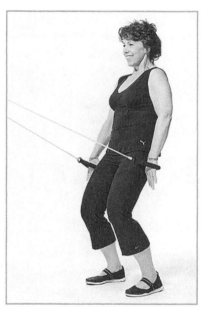

Start: Anchor the band securely at chest height. Facing the anchor point, hold the handles in each hand, with your hands extended forward at shoulder height, palms facing the floor, feet hip-width apart. Suck in your tummy and bend your knees as though you were sitting in a chair. At the same time, pull the handles down to your sides, keeping arms straight, palms facing back. Hold for 1 count and straighten up. Repeat for 15 reps.

Form: Hold your tummy tightly in for the entire set, breathing out as you lower and pull, inhaling as you rise to the start position. Keep elbows locked for the rep. Count 3 seconds to bend; hold for 1 count and then count 3 seconds to return to start.

As you get stronger, add a small jump in between each rep, as you straighten up to the start position.

Push-Ups

The push-up is the single-most effective exercise on the planet for overall fitness. It works the shoulders, chest, arms, upper back and abs. Your body weight provides most of the resistance, but we're going to add a bit more with the band to get that definition in your triceps that you crave. Don't get discouraged with this one. You are pressing your full body weight, which may be more than you like right now. As you get smaller and stronger, you'll be amazed at how well you do with push-ups.

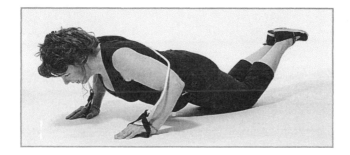

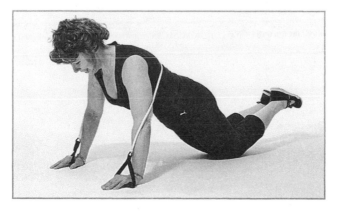

Start: Position the band across your shoulder blades with handles in each hand. Lie facedown with your hands at shoulder height, palms on the floor, holding the handles, just wider than shoulder-width, elbows bent. Suck in your tummy and press your body up in a straight line, keeping your knees on the floor. Your body should form a straight diagonal line from head to knees, the band tight. Hold for 1 count and then lower your body, leading with your chest, almost to the floor. Hold for 1 count and repeat for 15 reps.

Form: Hold your tummy tight for the whole set. Breathe out as you push up and inhale as you lower your body to the floor. Raise up as you count 3 seconds; hold for 1 count and then lower for a count of 3 seconds. Don't drop down or let your middle sag as you do the reps. It's better if you do fewer reps and do them right, building up to 15 over a couple of weeks.

As you get stronger, get off your knees. Press your whole body up in a straight line from head to toes, with just your palms and the balls of your feet on the floor.

Curls

This exercise works the biceps, giving them definition and tone. I love this exercise. I could do it all day and never, ever tire of it. No more flabby arms.

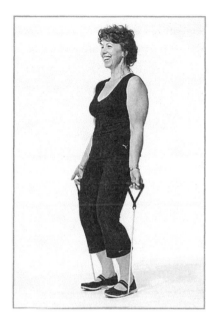 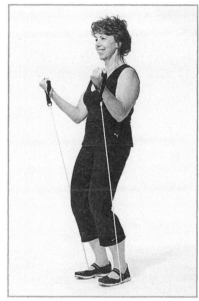

Start: Stand with your feet hip-width apart, knees soft, the band under your feet, pulled tight. Hold a handle in each hand, arms at your side, palms facing legs. Keeping your upper arms still, curl both hands toward your shoulders, squeezing your bicep as you pull up. Stop the curl about 20 degrees from your shoulders. Hold for 1 count, squeezing your biceps and lower to the start position. Repeat for 15 reps.

Form: Hold your tummy tight during the set. Breathe out as you curl and inhale as you lower your arms. As you curl, pretend that your elbows are glued to your side, so you isolate the bicep. Don't swing the curl or use your back. Curl up on a 3-second count; hold for 1 count and lower to a 3-second count. Don't let the band pull your arm down. Use the bicep; feel it contract. If the move is too hard at first, stand with your feet closer together to loosen the resistance of the band, widening your stance as you progress.

As you get stronger, add half-curls to the set. Curl from the bottom and stop the curl when your forearm is at 90 degrees. Hold for 1 count and lower. Repeat for 15 reps.

And as you get even stronger, you can add resistance by simply criss-crossing the band across your body (forming an *x*) and curling.

Kickback

You will grow to love the kickback, as you watch that flapping skin on the backs of your upper arms tighten and define. It's hard, but being able to go sleeveless is worth the work, I'd say.

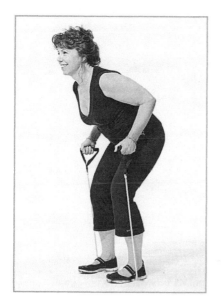 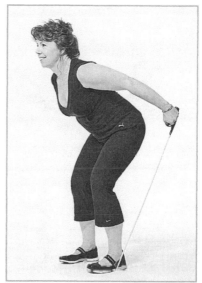

Start: Stand with feet just under hip-width apart, knees slightly bent. Place the band under your feet, a handle in each hand. Bend forward from hips, keeping your back flat until you are at a 45-degree angle, with upper arms by your sides, parallel to the floor. Bend your forearms to 90 degrees. With your tummy sucked in, press forearms back, straightening them, turning your palms to the ceiling. Hold for 1 count and return to start position. Repeat for 15 reps.

Form: Keep your tummy tight for the whole set. Breathe out as you press your forearms back and inhale as you return to the start position. Keep your arms close and tight to your body, so your arms are pressing straight back. You should feel your triceps (back upper arms) tighten. Press arms back for a 3-second count; hold for 1 count and lower to a 3-second count. Don't let the band pull your arms back. Resist so you work the triceps.

As you get stronger, place the band under your feet with some slack between your feet so you create greater resistance.

Recline Row

This exercise works your shoulders, arms, back and abs. This exercise creates the kind of gorgeous shoulders that love sleeveless shirts and dresses. And strength-building? Just wait and see.

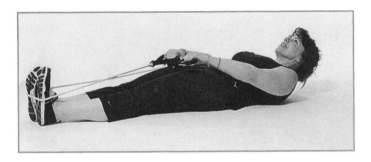

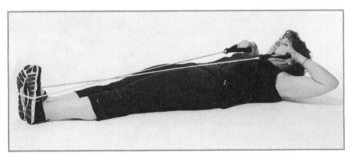

Start: Lie faceup with the band under your feet. Crisscross the band across your body and hold a handle in each hand. (The band will form an *x* across your body). Extend your arms toward your feet, palms down. Suck in your tummy and raise your head and shoulders off the floor. With shoulders lifted, pull hands toward your chest, bending elbows, keeping your hands close to your body. Your elbows will flare out to the sides. Pull as close to shoulder height as you can. Hold for 1 count and repeat for 15 reps.

Form: Keep your abs tight for the entire set. Breathe out as you pull your hands to your chest and inhale as you extend your arms toward your feet. Keep your head and shoulders raised, but don't place strain on your neck. When you raise your head, pretend that you have an apple under your chin. That will help you keep your head straight and the strain on your abs, not your neck. Pull up for a 3-second count; hold for 1 count and extend your hands toward your feet for a 3-second count.

As you get stronger, change this exercise to a standing row. It's the same exercise, but you are standing and pulling your hands up toward your shoulders. Standing makes for more resistance.

Thigh Press and Crunch

This compound move works your abs, lower back and thighs, particularly the inner thighs and "saddlebag" area. It's genius.

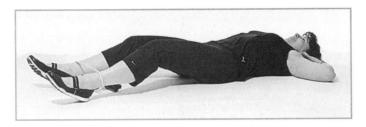

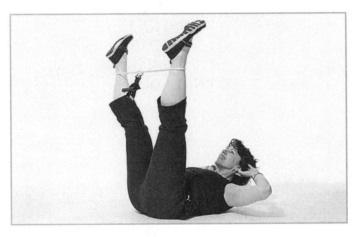

Start: Knot the band around your legs midway from knees to feet, with feet shoulder-width apart. Lie faceup, legs bent at the hips, straight in the air (90 degrees to the hips). Place your hands behind your head, elbows wide. Contract your abs, lifting your head and shoulders off the floor, keeping elbows wide. At the same time you crunch up, press your legs wide apart against the resistance of the band. Hold for 1 count and lower to the start. Repeat for 15 reps.

Form: Contract your abs for the entire set. As you lift into the crunch, pretend that there is an apple under your chin. This keeps your neck straight, preventing strain and keeping the stress on your abs. Keep your elbows wide as you crunch up; do not pull up with your arms on your neck. Pull up with your abs. Breathe out as you crunch up and press legs out. Inhale as you return to the start position. Crunch up and press out to a 3-second count; hold for 1 count and then return to the start for a 3-second count.

Leg Lift

This exercise works your butt, keeping it firm and preventing it from sagging south…or pulling it back up. It also works the backs of your thighs, creating shapely legs and great strength.

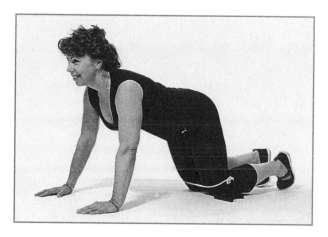

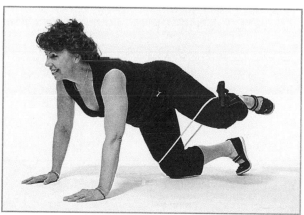

Start: Knot band securely around your mid thighs. Kneel on all fours (with a cushion under your knees if needed). Suck in your tummy and keep your back straight and flat. Lift your right leg out to the side as high as you can, trying for 90 degrees or hip height. Hold for 1 count and lower. Repeat for 15 reps and then repeat the set on the left leg.

Form: Make sure that your body is like a table when you are on all fours…back straight and flat, abs sucked in, legs and arms at 90 degrees from your body (hands directly under shoulders, knees under hips). Breathe out as you raise your leg and inhale as you lower it. Raise your leg to a 3-second count; hold for 1 count and lower it to a 3-second count.

As you get stronger, hold your leg at the top position and pulse quickly up and down for 8 counts before lowering to the floor. Repeat pulses in between each rep.

Bicycle

I saved the best for last. This classic exercise is the single-most effective exercise for your abs. It works all of them: upper, lower, obliques. It's hard, but it's perfect.

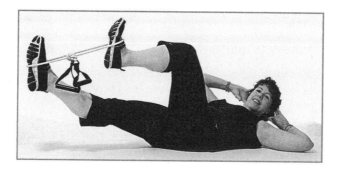

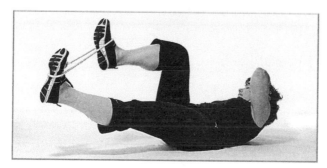

Start: Tie your band around your feet at the arches, with feet shoulder-width apart. Lie on your back with your legs bent to 90 degrees, feet flexed to hold the band in place, hands behind your head, elbows wide. Lift your head and shoulders off the floor, twisting your left elbow toward your right knee. At the same time, pull your right knee in as though trying to touch your elbow and knee. Then twist the right elbow toward the left knee, again pulling your left knee in toward the elbow, simulating the motion of your legs riding a bike, all the while twisting your upper body from side to side. Continue for 15 full reps (15 on each side).

Form: Contract your abs tightly for the entire set. Try to keep your elbows wide as you twist so that the strain is on your side abs (obliques) and not your neck. Breathe out as you twist and inhale as your body straightens before going into the alternate twist.

As you get stronger, add a second...and third set of reps.

THE FINAL MOVES

Your workout is complete and you feel great, maybe a bit spent, but great. But ah-ah-ah...not so fast. Don't forget to stretch. I close my workout with these simple stretches every time so that I stay loose—as we say at my gym.

And did I mention that these simple stretches can be done anytime, anywhere? Outside of your workout, taking a little "stretch break" can make you feel relaxed and alert, so enjoy them anytime!

Forward Bend

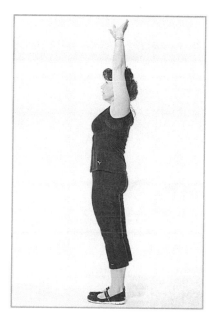 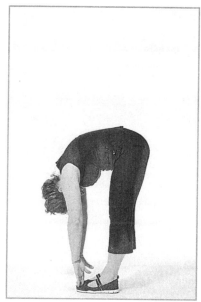

Stand with your feet together, hands and arms relaxed, hanging at your sides. As you inhale, raise your arms over your head, reaching hard for the ceiling. Exhale, dropping forward from your waist, letting your hands and arms move toward your toes. Allow the weight of your body to pull you into a comfortable stretch. Your knees can be slightly bent if it's more comfortable for you but a straight-legged bend is best. You want to stretch, not strain! Stay bent in this position for 3 breaths. Do not push or bounce. You should not feel pain, just a stretch of the backs of your thighs, calves and lower back. Repeat this stretch 3 to 5 times.

Leg Stretch

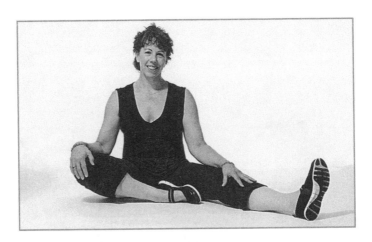

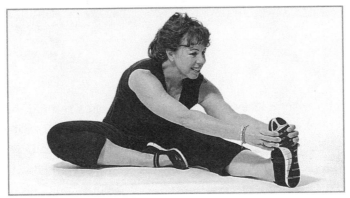

Sit on the floor (on a mat, if you want your butt cushioned) with your legs straight out in front of you. Bend your right leg and place the sole of your foot on your upper inner left thigh and lower your knee to the floor, or as close as you can without pain. Keep your left leg straight, the foot flexed and pointing toward the ceiling, and press your knee into the floor. Sit up straight. Inhale and raise your arms over your head. Exhale and as you reach toward your left foot, reaching for the toes. Hold for 3 breaths. Sit up, and place your left hand on your bent right knee and twist to the right, stretching your back. Hold for 3 breaths. Repeat this same sequence on the left side.

Remember that stretching should open and relax your body, not hurt, so while you want to push the stretch a bit, don't push until you feel pain. You should feel the pull of your muscles as they open naturally, but it should not be agonizing. Stretching is gentle, not crazy, and you will progress into deeper and deeper stretches if you stretch regularly.

Veganomics is about changing the way you think about your all aspects of your health but there's more to life than just you. When you commit to change your thinking, it's not limited to your personal well-being. A very wise teacher once told me that all we need to do to clean up the environment is to clean up our own internal environment. As he patted his tummy, said if "that" was "clean," then the world would follow—and he spread his arms wide. He went on to explain that once your body is healthy and vital, organs functioning well, blood strong and clean, you can no longer tolerate an environment that isn't as healthy as you are, so it changes by your actions, resulting in a cleaner, healthier world.

Once you get your own house in order, there are lots of things that you can do to make the world around you a more hospitable place. Next up, see what you can do to change the world, one lightbulb at a time.

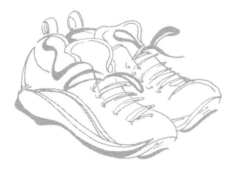

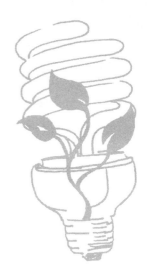

8

This Crazy Vegan Lifestyle

All across the world, in every kind of environment and region known to man, increasingly dangerous weather patterns and devastating storms are abruptly putting an end to the long-running debate over whether or not climate change is real. Not only is it real, it's here and its effects are giving rise to a frighteningly new global phenomenon— the man-made natural disaster. —BARACK OBAMA

Lifestyle: Doesn't the very word signal that this is the point in the book for the airy-fairy, touchy-feely, new age sensitive stuff? Sorry. That's not *my* style. What I want you to get out of this book is good, solid information that you can use to become a fitter, healthier human who leaves a lighter footprint on the planet. The fact that you will also be happier, kinder and more compassionate just comes along with the package because living a vegan life will change you in ways that you might never have imagined, ways that encompass more than your physical body. And I guarantee that you'll love those changes.

When I was first studying macrobiotics under the famed teacher Michio Kushi, my fellow students and I were bemoaning the plight of the environment and trying to figure out what we could do about it. Kushi said that we didn't need to organize rallies or make signs to protest. Rather, all we needed to do was teach people about food and how to eat. His theory was that as we ate foods appropriate to humans, we would find ourselves in harmony with the environment around us. As more and more people ate well and became naturally more fit, the improvement in the environment would follow because as we'd learn to live as natural humans and we'd have it no other way.

Over the past twenty-five years as I've changed my food and my life, I have become much more conscious of the impact that my choices make on the planet. While my personal journey might have started with something as simple as giving up paper towels and paper napkins, it's certainly progressed since then. (I've also been rethinking that concept we call "progress"…) There's no denying that I still make a footprint, but I make every effort to make that it smaller and lighter. I do fly commercially for much of my work. I do have to drive for my work as well. But as I grow in this lifestyle (yes, I still grow…), I discover new and wonderful ways to lessen my impact on the environment and even try to make it a little better for my being here.

You may think that it's a no-brainer to live consciously and be kind to the planet. Or you may be one of the millions of people who have no idea of the impact you are making or how to make greener choices in life. As you change your thinking and actions about food you will be more awake to the bigger problems we humans create for our planet. You will, as I do, wonder how people can call themselves environmentalists and still sit down to steak dinners—an inconvenient truth to be sure, but truth nonetheless.

Choosing to live a sustainable lifestyle begins in the kitchen, extends throughout your home, into the garden, and into the community. Like the ripples from a pebble thrown into water, each choice you make has an impact that is felt around the world. It will take the effort of each and every one of us to alter the collision course that we are currently on, but if you want to ensure a future for generations to come, the time to act is now.

I am not saying that you have to give up your car completely (unless it's one of those gas-guzzling, debt-creating, mammoth vehicles) or that you have to live "off the grid," but you do have to make choices that let the rest of the world see that you are awake! You can begin with small changes and see where they lead you—just like with your food. But the *one* thing you can't do is *nothing*. The good news is that once you have cleaned up your diet, the rest just follows. It's like your consciousness grows with each healthy meal, with each exercise session. You want clean water, clean air, pure food and you are willing to do what it takes to get it.

But if you're lost and have no idea where to begin, I've got you covered. The things that you can do right now will amaze you and will change our fragile environment for the better and forever.

Your Home

I know you want to save the planet, but some of the following ideas can also help you save money. Now I know I have your attention!

Life ... Unplugged

We all know that we should turn off the lights in rooms where there are no people, right? I say, take it a step further. Shut down your computer and printer, instead of leaving them on "hibernate," idling away energy when not in use. When you leave the house for the day, take a second and unplug fans, televisions, stereos, the coffee machine, the toaster. It may be a bother at first, but when you see those few dollars' savings on your electric bill, you ... and the planet will have won a small battle. And if you have kids, it's a great chore for them in the morning. Unplugging the appliances before leaving for school creates a consciousness in them that they will take with them through life. Everyone will get used to the new routine in just a few days.

When you are on the market for new appliances, always look for the energy-efficient models with fewer "bells and whistles." Do you really need a fridge with a tv set in the door? Even an icemaker uses more energy than you might think.

For your appliances already in use, take a few minutes to make them more efficient. Clean the filters on your air conditioners, and insulate water heaters and keep up with the simple maintenance needed to keep them running efficiently. You save money, your appliances will last longer, you take a bit of the burden off the planet.

Light Up the World—Responsibly

Don't you dare tell me that you won't switch to fluorescent bulbs because you think they are like the ones buzzing and flickering and throwing off that institutional light that reminds you of old hospitals and prisons! There's real progress on this front; manufacturers have responded to both our environmental and aesthetic sensibilities with bulbs that are, shall we say, more flattering. Look for high "lumens," not watts for brighter light and read the labels for indications of color renderings that give warmer light, more like the incandescence that you are used to. (The prices are coming way down on these long-lasting, energy-efficient bulbs, so you win again.)

If you think that lightbulbs are no big deal, think again. If every American household replaced their five most-used light fixtures with florescent bulbs, this country would save $8 billion in energy costs. There's a lot of Mother Nature preserved in that number.

Get Cozy

You've heard these ones a million times, but just in case you missed it: Insulate your home to conserve the energy used to cool and heat it. Block up any drafts or leaks in windows or doors. Ceiling fans can help you to use less air conditioning in the heat of summer and can also help to keep heated air from being trapped near the ceiling, so you use less energy to heat and cool your home. Just setting your thermostat to 66 degrees in the winter and 78 degrees in the summer will save you hundreds of dollars in energy costs and countless resources.

Power Up—or Down

In many areas, you can now opt to buy renewable energy from your local power company. Wind power, methane and the sun are now being tapped by large energy companies to provide green sources of electricity.

How do you know if you have an enlightened power company? (Sorry, I couldn't resist that one…) Check out the Green Power Network's map of the United States for information on utility companies that are working for the environment as well as for you.

Or you can move to Austin, Texas, which is not only famous for its music scene but is also a consistent national leader in using "green power."

Renewable energy may cost a few cents more each month but you help support its use if you opt for it when it's offered by your local power company—and save lots more than just a few pennies in the end.

Water: Save a Little, Save a Lot

When I was a kid, my mother would stand over us at the sink while we brushed our teeth. Of course, her main goal was to make sure that we actually brushed our teeth. But she also reminded us to turn off the water while we brushed. I can hear her voice in my head to this day, when I brush my teeth. "Do you think that there is an infinite amount of water on this earth?" she would ask. Yes, I would think. But she was right. So I learned to conserve water, which I still do to this day.

Check this out: The water heater in the average American home is the second-largest consumer of energy, right behind heating. Turning the thermostat on the water heater down to 120 degrees will give you plenty of hot water for your needs and save energy. You can also install a timer on your water heater so that it's working only at the times when you are most likely to use it. There's no need to use the energy to heat water while the house is sleeping. The timer can switch the heater on an hour before you get up and it's ready to go! You can even go to the step of installing a pump that recycles the water you use, filtering it so you use less water—saving up to 21,000 gallons each year for an average family of four people.

As much as you love long, hot showers, those leisurely streams of water coursing over you are luxuries this planet can't afford. A quick five-minute shower is wiser for the planet and your wallet, but if you like the idea of a long, relaxing steam in hot water, try a bath instead. You use much less water that way. You can also install low-flow showerheads, which prevents heavy torrents of water from flowing but still provides plenty of power to clean up. And of course, you are using natural soaps to clean your bodies, right? They are better for the health of your skin and our waterways.

In the kitchen, fill the sink or a basin with water and wash the dishes. Then rinse. Constant running of water to do dishes wastes gallons and gallons of this precious resource. Turn off the water while scrubbing pots and pans. Dishwashers used to be total water hogs, but the newer models can actually save water and energy, with some using only four gallons of water for a full load of dishes. Check them out.

Turn up the temperature in the fridge a little. It doesn't have to be like the North Pole in there to keep food fresh. And use ice trays for your ice cubes instead of water-guzzling ice makers.

And then there's laundry. Wash only full loads, using warm water with a cold rinse. That will get your clothes plenty clean. And since we're on the subject of laundry, use only those soaps that are kind to the planet. There are so many good options now, some available right in your supermarket. Your clean laundry should not result in polluted waterways.

And don't forget to turn off the water when you're shaving or brushing your teeth. Happy, Mom?

Cleaning Your House

Speaking of Mom and water, I know that she'd be happy to hear that I love to clean. I think it's genetically wired into my ancestry. To me, there is nothing more gratifying than surveying my sparkling-clean house. I have worked up a sweat, to be sure, but wow! Whether you share my passion or have some help in the housecleaning department, there is no excuse for polluting the planet—or endangering your own health—as you spit-shine your countertops and floors.

Even the EPA is on board with this one, issuing a statement that 50% of all chronic illnesses can be traced to indoor pollution, most of which comes from ordinary household cleaners. Interestingly, they believe that indoor pollution is about ten times more toxic for us than the outside poisons we worry so much about.

My own experience has been that most household products don't really warn of the dangers of the chemicals in their products or tell us that the disposal of these chemicals is toxic to our waterways.

Here are some of the villains to look for when you are reading labels in the cleaning aisle of your supermarket:

Petroleum is used as a solvent for cleaners. You can recognize this one in the cleaners that evaporate quickly and leave no streaks or marks behind. The toxic fumes are delightful, too.

Phosphates are compounds used in commercial laundry detergents, which contribute to serious water pollution.

Butane and *pentane* are just two of the chemicals used in those smelly air sprays. Before you spritz your home to create the scent of wildflowers, consider this: The organic chemicals in those sprays contribute to the formation of ozone in the lower atmosphere, a major contributor to air pollution, especially in cities. Buy fresh, fragrant flowers instead. You get a lovely perfume in the air and your home is prettier.

Chlorine is used in bleach to create the whitest whites and to sanitize surfaces, but it is a major contributor to water pollution, killing off lots of wildlife and creating fish that are too toxic to eat.

So are you meant to have a less-than-sparkling home, dull whites and smelly rooms? Of course not. There are so many natural alternatives to clean your home and you won't be polluting the air and water or leaving behind a chemical haze when you wipe your counters.

You just have to rethink *how* you clean. You can purchase some of the many products that have been created to make cleaning more green, from glass cleaner to laundry detergent to liquid dish soap, toilet cleaner and floor polish. If you need to clean it, there is a natural product available.

Some of the natural cleaners can be more expensive, but don't worry. There are items that are probably already in your pantry that clean so well, even Martha Stewart would be impressed.

Humble baking soda is one of the stars of my cleaning tools. Sure, you all know that you can place a box in the fridge to absorb food odors. But did you know that you can use it to clean and deodorize other bits of the house? It softens water, which improves sudsing, so you can use less soap. It's great for scouring *anything*. You can place about a half cup of it in the bottom of a trash can to keep odors at bay. Here's my favorite: It is the greatest fabric softener I have ever used. And if you dissolve it into a thick paste with a little water, it makes a great silver polish.

Borax, found in the laundry aisle of your grocery, is a great deodorizer and a fabulous cleanser when mixed with soap. Great for disinfecting, borax also works very well as a color enhancer, brightening coloreds and whitening whites, so no bleach is necessary and you still have bright, clean laundry.

Before I discovered green cleaning products, I had no idea what washing powder was or did. You can find it in the laundry section of your market. It is the best natural degreaser and stain remover I have found. You know all those stain removers that exist? You spray them on or rub them in with a brush. Well, your laundry may be stain-free, but these products are seriously toxic for the environment. Simple washing powder (called precisely that) removes stains as well as anything you can "shout out."

White vinegar is big favorite in my house. I use it for everything: cleaning and freshening surfaces (including my hardwood floors), to cut grease and remove stains (even from carpets), to clean drains and as a fabric softener. You can even use it straight up to clean chrome surfaces to a spitshine sparkle.

On the occasions that I need to clean my oven, I use simple everyday ammonia to get the job done. It works beautifully. I'm supposed to tell you not to mix it with bleach when cleaning, but since you won't be using bleach anymore, that warning is not needed, right?

I love to mix lemon juice with a touch of vegetable oil to polish any unwaxed wood surface in the house. A brisk buff brings out the shine and you get stronger, leaner arms in the process of buffing.

Also remember to open the windows to create a bit of ventilation in your home and to help freshen the air. Even on the coldest days, just ten minutes of fresh air in the house changes the environment completely. Try it!

Junk Mail

Junk mail is aptly named. It adds clutter to our lives—and just think of all the trees that are sacrificed for the fourteen Victoria's Secret catalogs that you get every week. Rethink: Log on to www.catalogchoice.org and follow the simple steps to rid your mailbox of a lot of junk.

PLANT SOMETHING…ANYTHING!

Garden projects, planting trees, creating or contributing to community gardens, working with schools or your neighborhood to create edible gardens offer gratification like nothing else you can do in nature. And if that's not enough for you, consider this: You get some much-needed exercise when you plant. You work up a sweat, so your body's stronger and healthier and, because you planted something, the planet's stronger and healthier, too.

Trees are amazing creatures, each with a personality all its own. And boy, do they love us! Trading carbon dioxide for oxygen, we breathe easier having trees around. They shade our homes, allowing for less energy use in the summer heat. They increase the real estate value of our homes. Birds and squirrels love to live in them. They add beauty and serenity to any neighborhood.

A garden is a place of nourishment for our bodies and souls. Flowers, herbs, vegetables and fruits all serve as signs that life is a beautiful and precious thing. If you want to reconnect to your natural self, plant a garden and watch it thrive under your care. As the garden matures and the flowers burst with color, fragrant with their perfume, you will be intoxicated by life itself. Make a salad from your own garden greens and you will feel the life inside you. It's hard to feel depressed when you are out in the garden, coaxing life from plants with your gentle touch. From windowboxes to container gardens to small farms, planting is life.

If getting your fingers in the dirt is just not your cup of decaf tea, buy a tree. You heard me: Buy a tree. Many organizations offer the chance to buy trees to be planted in areas of the world devastated by industry or natural disaster. You can help to bring those places back to life with your donation.

Get involved by donating your time and/or money to a community or school garden. I work as a volunteer in one of my city's high schools and when we instituted our edible garden program, no one was certain we would succeed, even me. But as the school year went on, I noticed a light in my students' eyes as they watched their seeds break through the soil. I watched these tough city kids nurture lettuce, peas and basil to tender maturity with a pride I had not seen in them before.

Want some serious self-satisfaction in life? Plant something and watch it grow!

The Grass Is Always Greener—or Is It?

More than 31% of the water used in this country waters lawns. Now, I would never tell you to get rid of the glorious green that carpets your property, but look around for better ways to irrigate it. There are new innovations that use less water and still maintain the vivid green you love. Oh, and skip the fertilizer on your grass, unless it's natural. All those chemicals sprayed on lawns pollute the air and water and with natural options being just as effective, why go the chemical route?

Better yet, find alternatives to grass . . . There are many sources to help you, including the earth-friendly folks at www.eartheasy.com.

Recycle . . . More and More and More

Recycling is certainly a popular topic nowadays—and you probably think you've heard everything there is to say about it. But there's so much more than using canvas totes at the grocery store instead of "plastic or paper," although it's a good place to start. Take all your plastic bags back to the supermarket and use them again or drop them into the recycling bin that most markets have at the door. Use those hip-looking canvas totes to transport your groceries—it's a great way to advertise your commitment.

And here's a bunch of other ideas that might not have occurred to you:

Many participating mechanic shops recycle motor oil, antifreeze, tires and car batteries. Do some research and find out who they are and give your business to them…or at least recycle with them.

Buy only greeting cards and note pads made from recycled paper. They are so lovely and well designed. You will be sending your heartfelt thoughts to your loved ones and the planet.

Donate your old cell phones, electronics and computers to charities that will repair and recycle them. Many cell companies give the phones to shelters for abused women so they have access to emergency aid. Cars can be donated to various charities for repair and resale. You get a tax write-off and the planet has one less car in the junk pile.

Compost your food scraps and use them to feed your garden (or your neighbor's, if you don't have your own patch of heaven) and let the cut grass clippings lay on the lawn. They are a great source of nutrients to keep your grass healthy and vividly green.

Donate your clothing, shoes, coats and handbags to shelters, thrift stores or charities that aid disaster victims. There's no reason to throw those peacoats, slingbacks or shoulder bags in the trash just because you are "over" them. If they are in good condition and clean, lots of people can get lots of use out of them before they need to hit the trash pile.

Just about anything and everything that you own can be reused or repurposed. Once man's junk is, as they say, another's treasure. There are so many people who have so little and many who have so much. Your excess can become someone's salvation. The more we can recycle, the less we burden the landfill with our trashed belongings—and the more we share the wealth, the richer we all will be.

It's time to think outside the box on recycling…literally.

Skip the Package

We simply must remove some of the layers that come between us and the products we consume. Think about it. You buy a bit of stuff. The stuff is in a plastic pouch, inside a plastic mold, maybe a blister pack, inside a paper sleeve or on a paper card. You purchase the stuff, which is placed in a bag for you to take home. Wow! We buy razor blades, toothbrushes, mascara, snacks, cookies, cereal, soda, chewing gum... all in so much packaging that our landfills are choked with this trash, which will take decades to decompose, if ever. The fact that you can never get the silly packages open should be enough to inspire you to look for something simpler.

It's easy to choose products that use less packaging, if you look. Certainly packaging is necessary for some things. Certainly there are sanitation issues that make packaging necessary in some cases. There's no need to be obsessive, but we have moved a long way from natural. Use your head. Refill where you can. Buy in bulk—things like grains and beans are much more economical when you reject all the little pouches inside packages. Buy a head of lettuce instead of salad in a bag. Purchase carrots loose, if you can. You get the idea.

Park It

With gas prices skyrocketing and no substantial relief in sight, everyone knows that there has to be a better way. There is, but it requires new thinking.

Alternative fuel sources are certainly the way of the future, but the planet—and your wallet—need relief now. How any single person can drive a Hummer or any oversized SUV that's not a hybrid is completely beyond my comprehension. It seems unconscionable to me to burn resources at that level to drive to the mall or supermarket. I truly don't buy the whole "these cars make us feel safer" argument either. Do we live in war zones? I apologize if I have insulted anyone who drives one, but you might want to rethink your transportation.

Ranting aside, simply driving less than twenty miles a day can add up to more than $2,000 in energy costs. Most cities have decent mass transit systems, trains, buses, suburban routes to the city. There are lots of options to driving. And there's always the old reliable idea of carpooling.

Ride a bike to work; walk for errands…or jog. You'll be fitter, richer and kinder to the planet. I know that leaving the car at home every day is not an option for many people. But if you could replace even two car trips a week, you'll save money and energy. Or you could just drive smarter. Combine several errands in one trip, mapping a route that saves miles. Group appointments into one day; shop near your home for essentials; drive the speed limit.

And walk, walk, walk…

Live It—a Little at a Time

If you live greener, people can't help but notice. Everyone wants to do better. Everyone is worried about this fragile planet of ours. Everyone is shocked by the loser who throws soda cans and cigarettes out of their car windows. We all want to make a difference, contributing to the health of the planet. We can all learn from each other, if we just pay attention. Start out small and just watch how quickly the little steps lead to the bigger strides toward living green.

Start with the small things in life, changes you can live with. Pick your battles. For me, it began with paper products. I decided that I could live without paper towels a long time ago and just stopped buying them. I keep a bin of rags under the sink and just add them to my loads of laundry. From there, we stopped buying paper napkins. I invested in simple cotton napkins, which launder easily. Over the years, our use of paper products has been reduced to only toilet tissue. And life is no more complicated, no more work than before. We wash and reuse produce bags and plastic resealable bags (it takes us about three years to go through a box). We put filters on all our faucets, which power down the use of water. From paper products, the "greening" of our home grew and grew…from composting to recycling things we no longer use. We are pretty happy with the footprint that our day-to-day living leaves behind, but are always looking for ways to do better.

Remember that awareness is the first step toward action. It's all about changing the way we think about the planet, recycling, buying responsibly, supporting the good guys and the worthy causes and becoming a very powerful part of the solution.

Come Green with Me

Obviously, I have my ideas on being greener, but I am sure that there are so many things that I have not considered.

One of the best ways to "green" the world is by spreading the word. Talk to each other and share ideas. What works and what doesn't in the day-to-day chaos of life?

Head on over to www.christinacooks.com and look for my blog. I'm there talking about all sorts of things fitness, health, food, and the environment. Join our forum and share your thoughts . . . and read what other people are saying.

I can't wait to hear from you!

Resource Guide

One of the most common questions I am asked is how do I know everything that I know? Well, the short answer is that I have been doing what I do for a long time and I read everything.

You can't be expected to have all the answers at your fingertips unless, like me, it is your living. So to make your crazy vegan life easier, here is a list of the resources I use the most when I want to find the truth behind the spin, when I am looking for solid, credible information and when I just want to learn more.

www.christinacooks.com (obviously...)
Vegan recipes, information and links to people of like mind.

www.christinapirello.org
The website for my education initiative dedicated to community outreach, in-school education about food and health, legislative efforts, work with farms and scholarship programs.

www.truefoodnow.org
The truth behind labeling and a comprehensive list on all the players.

www.centerforfoodsafety.org
The Center for Food Safety works to protect human health and the environment through information and action.

www.pcrm.org
The Physicians' Committee for Responsible Medicine is a wealth of information on health-related issues, diet concerns and making the transition to vegan eating easier.

www.organicconsumers.org

The Organic Consumers Association offers comprehensive information, links, current news and campaigns to promote change.

www.sustainabletable.org

The Sustainable Table created this website to help consumers understand our food supply, alternatives to commercial foods and viable environmental solutions to food production.

www.transfairusa.org

A website dedicated to the education and promotion of Fair Trade, a way of producing food that ensures that farmers receive fair prices for their products and other economic considerations so that they can survive. Look for their logo on coffee, chocolate, vanilla and other exotics to make a lighter footprint and to support small farms.

www.safecosmetics.org

A coalition of environmental and public health groups dedicated to protecting the health and welfare of the consuming public and workers of the personal care industry.

www.habitat.org

Habitat for Humanity not only builds houses in underserved and disaster areas of the world, but they accept used building supplies like paint and wood. They will also accept motor vehicles as donations (as do many others, but I love these guys). You get to help and recycle some of the most difficult items to recycle.

www.organic-center.org

An organization dedicated to creating a credible and easy-to-understand clearinghouse for information on organics, as well as promoting the use of organic methods in all walks of life.

www.cspinet.org

The Center for Science in the Public Interest, while controversial, is a no-nonsense site dedicated to advocacy for nutrition, food safety, sound science and policy. Their Nutrition Action Newsletter is great.

www.vrg.org

The Vegetarian Resource Group is a website dedicated to nutrition, recipes, meal plans and lots of information on living green and vegan.

www.chooseveg.com

A more radical vegan website with information on animal welfare, nutrition and the environment.

www.ota.com

The Organic Trade Association delivers information on organic standards, public policy and labeling issues.

www.chefsforhumanity.org

A nonprofit organization dedicated to eliminating world hunger and poor nutrition in schools.

www.greenpeace.org

The world's most effective environmental activist group, dedicated to issues of climate change, saving our ancient forests, toxic waste and other health concerns.

www.peta.org

The People for the Ethical Treatment of Animals offers a wealth of vegan-related information.

www.howstuffworks.com

To learn, well, how stuff works.

Acknowledgments

Oy, as I often say. It seems that the longer I work on my chosen path, the more people I meet along the way who deserve my deepest gratitude. I am humbled by those who surround me and support me; without them, I would do much less in this world.

John Duff, who has toiled as my publisher for more than ten years, is without a doubt one of the wisest and most amazing men I have had the pleasure to know. To work with him is a dream. Over the years, I have grown comfortable enough to tell him my wildest ideas and he knows me well enough to draw me back from what he calls "woo-woo land" when I need it. Thanks, John, for the years of support and confidence and friendship.

To Charles and Craig and Jeanette and everyone else at the Penguin Group for all that you do to support the work I do…thanks so much.

And there are my girls…that tiny group of powerful women friends who grace my life with their presence. Friendship is a small word for what they give. They are my family, my rocks and my sanity savers. So to Mary, Tina, Michele, Gayle, Sue and Cynthia, I love you for the blessings you bring to my life.

To the men who grace my life, Don, Richard, Larry, Robert (the other one), Will, David, Steve, Kevin and my sweet Dennis; thanks for being the men you are. You are the reasons I love men so much. If all women had men like you in their lives, there would be no male bashing because in you, women would see the true glory of men.

Anthony Molino and Al Richezza changed my life, from the standpoint of fitness. There is no way to put into words the gratitude I feel each and every time I achieve another fitness goal, complete a hard workout, cross a race finish line…or simply lift a heavy grocery sack without effort or get through my days with strength and grace. You have both brought gifts to my life that I thought were out of reach. Thanks for pushing me so hard.

Michio Kushi was my first teacher in natural living. When Robert introduced me to macrobiotics, I discovered your teaching and philosophy. I was blessed with the opportunity to study with you personally, and my understanding of food and its power (limited though it remains) is a result of what you showed me. No matter what I learn from other people and studies, I seem to always come back to the wisdom you passed on to me so many years ago. Thanks for your infinite generosity with your knowledge, your even more infinite patience with my slow understanding and your unfailing support for my work.

To all my students and recipe guinea pigs…thanks for all that you teach me. I love each and every one of you for all you have brought to my world.

My husband, Robert, is the finest man I know. His love is unconditional; his patience without end and his vision nothing less than magical. He has taken my life to places I could not imagine and we have loved every moment of our lives together. I said it best on the night I won the Emmy Award for *Christina Cooks*. I stood on the podium, praying that I would not trip down the steps. I remember saying only this: "Honey, you keep having the visions and I'll keep showing up." I love you, baby.

Index